T0305001

Resounding praise for
OESTROGEN MATTERS

"How could one flawed scientific conclusion become a persuasive juggernaut that changed the practice of women's health worldwide? In their fascinating account, Bluming and Tavris challenge that conclusion and unpack the reasons for its remarkable impact."
—Robert B. Cialdini, PhD, author of *Influence* and *Pre-Suasion*

"This is such an important book, I want to do all I can to encourage every woman to read it. Groundbreaking and carefully researched, *Oestrogen Matters* provides essential information about the many benefits of oestrogen at menopause and even after a diagnosis of breast cancer. It reveals the misinterpretation of study results that led women (and their doctors) to have unwarranted concerns about oestrogen use. The thoughtful information presented here will help women feel more comfortable taking oestrogen, leading to healthier, longer lives for many."
—Patricia T. Kelly, PhD, specialist in cancer risk assessment and author of *Assessing Your True Risk of Breast Cancer*

"Given breast cancer's substantial morbidity, mortality, emotional toll, and the vast consequences of its treatment, this frontal salvo on the conventional wisdom of oestrogen use is refreshing and welcome. The book will stir a lively debate about the merits of decades of existing clinical research on oestrogens and help reframe the way clinicians and patients view the trade-off between the benefits and risks of hormone therapy."
—Jerome P. Kassirer, MD, distinguished professor, Tufts University School of Medicine, and former editor in chief, *New England Journal of Medicine*

"Having spent over two decades advancing women's health, I was appalled by the Women's Health Initiative's efforts to sensationalize and distort their own findings to promote an anti-hormone-therapy agenda. I hope *Oestrogen Matters* draws enough attention to counter the fears and misinformation about HRT that so many women, and their physicians, still hold."

—Phyllis Greenberger, MSW, former president and CEO of the Society for Women's Health Research

"This book is long overdue, and I salute the authors for their courage and effort (and their clear, witty writing). I believe it is an ethical imperative for all clinicians who treat women in menopause or women with breast cancer to alert their patients to this book."

—Michael Baum, MD, Visiting Professor of Medical Humanities, University College London

"Bluming and Tavris tell oestrogen's story in a way that is both accessible to the general public and appropriate for professionals. This book is an exhaustively researched and meticulously reasoned vindication of HRT. Very enlightening!"

—Harriet Hall, MD, editor, *Science-Based Medicine*

"*Oestrogen Matters* unravels the intricate web of science, medicine, and gender politics surrounding oestrogen therapy. In their unflinching exploration, with meticulous research and a fearless examination of medical dogma, Drs. Bluming and Tavris illuminate the complex terrain of oestrogen's effects on women's health. The result is an excellent resource for women."

—Peter Attia, MD, author of *Outlive: The Science and Art of Longevity*

Oestrogen
Matters

Oestrogen Matters

Why Taking Hormones in Menopause
Can Improve and Lengthen Women's
Lives—Without Raising the
Risk of Breast Cancer

The book that changed the conversation about HRT

Revised and Updated

Avrum Bluming, MD, and Carol Tavris, PhD

PIATKUS

PIATKUS

First published in the US in 2018 by Little, Brown Spark, Hachette Book Group, Inc.
This revised edition published in Great Britain in 2024 by Piatkus

5 7 9 10 8 6 4

A CIP catalogue record for this book
is available from the British Library.

ISBN 978-0-349-44347-8

Printed and bound in Great Britain by
Clays Ltd, Elcograf S.p.A

Papers used by Piatkus are from well-managed forests
and other responsible sources.

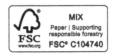

Piatkus
An imprint of
Little, Brown Book Group
Carmelite House
50 Victoria Embankment
London EC4Y 0DZ

The authorised representative
in the EEA is
Hachette Ireland
8 Castlecourt Centre
Dublin 15, D15 XTP3, Ireland
(email: info@hbgi.ie)

An Hachette UK Company
www.hachette.co.uk
www.littlebrown.co.uk

NOTE: The publishers of this edition have chosen to use the word 'oestrogen', rather than the
US version 'estrogen', as it is more familiar to readers outside the United States.

*To my patients, whose trust, courage, understanding, and
cooperation made my research possible,
and to my wife, Martha, who makes anything possible.
—Avrum Bluming*

Contents

You don't run against logic. You run against people who can't change their minds.
— Grace Murray Hopper, Navy rear admiral, mathematician, and pioneer in computer programming

Always underestimate the public's knowledge of a subject, but never underestimate their intelligence.
— Sir Denis Forman, founding member of the Grenada Television franchise (UK)

Oestrogen
Matters

Introduction

Who Killed HRT?

Avrum's story:

Not long ago I received an email from a woman who was agonizing over suspicious findings on her breast ultrasound. Her mammogram had shown a probable cyst, so the radiologist had ordered the ultrasound, and the results suggested a malignancy. The woman, whom I didn't know but who had been referred to me by a mutual friend, wrote that she was "freaking out," feeling hopeless, and already anticipating a total mastectomy; she added that if she could have her whole torso surgically removed, she would. This woman was a 50-year-old university professor of experimental psychology, yet she was completely panicked even before a biopsy had been performed.

I am profoundly aware of the fear that accompanies even a suspicion of a breast cancer diagnosis. I have been a medical oncologist for many decades, and about 60 percent of my practice is devoted to the study and treatment of breast cancer. In 1988, at the age of

45, my wife, Martha, was diagnosed with breast cancer. She had found a small nodule that seemed benign but nonetheless warranted removal, and I vividly remember my fear when the surgeon told us, "I'm sorry—it's a carcinoma." I felt as though I had been walking along a rocky path on a high mountain holding Martha's hand, and we had suddenly lost our footing. Two days later, the surgeon told us almost casually that the nodes he'd sent for biopsy when he removed the tumor appeared completely normal. I regained my balance. Whatever else might turn up, there was a good chance that Martha would be cured.

After Martha's lumpectomy, she received radiotherapy and chemotherapy, which pushed her into menopause; severe symptoms began and continued unabated. She didn't complain, understanding better than I what women were expected to tolerate in that era as part of the "change of life." But she was most definitely suffering. For years, the women under my care had reported a variety of the same symptoms: hot flushes, loss of sexual desire, painful intercourse because of vaginal dryness, difficulty sleeping, severe bladder pain, heart palpitations, unexplained and uncharacteristic anxiety attacks, difficulty concentrating, and—the thing that especially bothered Martha—fuzzy thinking, such as trouble remembering phone numbers and following the plot of a book.

And so I delved more systematically into the world of menopausal symptoms and their treatment. At the time, the uncontested most effective treatment for these symptoms was oestrogen. Because oestrogen therapy alone is associated with an increased risk of endometrial cancer (cancer of the lining of the uterus), women who still have a uterus are given hormone replacement therapy (HRT)—oestrogen plus progesterone—which provides the benefits of oestrogen without the increased risk of endometrial cancer. (Today, many physicians and laypeople dislike the word *replacement* and prefer to use the term *menopausal hormone therapy* or the even vaguer term *hormone therapy*. We will stay with *hormone replacement therapy*—HRT—in this book because it refers explicitly to the combination of the two hormones.) Martha asked me about prescribing oestrogen for her. Many of my menopausal patients who had been treated for breast cancer over the years had requested the same thing. They complained of severe impairment in the quality of their lives that they hoped oestrogen would alleviate. I had always advised against it because of the prevalent concern that oestrogen might increase the risk of cancer recurrence. (We discuss the evidence that currently disputes this belief in chapters 2 and 3.)

But motivated by Martha's unhappiness over her brain fog, I scoured the medical literature to see what I could find out about oestrogen's benefits and risks. It was an eye-opening journey. I began a study to evaluate the risks and benefits of HRT in breast cancer survivors (including Martha). With the women's full knowledge and consent, I administered the therapy and followed them over the years. The results of that study and many others I unearthed led me to write this book.

By the early 1990s, researchers had fifty years of well-documented evidence showing oestrogen's benefits. Oestrogen not only successfully controlled menopausal symptoms in most women but also significantly reduced the risks of heart disease, hip fractures, colon cancer, and Alzheimer's. A 1991 *New England Journal of Medicine* editorial titled "Uncertainty about Postmenopausal Oestrogen: Time for Action, Not Debate" reported a 40 to 50 percent reduction in atherosclerotic heart disease, which is responsible for the deaths of more than seven times as many American women as breast cancer.[1] The long-running Framingham study reported a 50 percent drop in osteoporosis-associated hip fractures, which were linked to as many deaths every year as breast cancer. Two studies, one from the University of Wisconsin and one from the American Cancer Society, reported a 50 percent decrease in the risk of developing or dying of colon cancer. Among women with no history of breast cancer, oestrogen did not increase the risk of developing it, even for women who took oestrogen for 10 to 15 years. Most notably, women taking oestrogen lived longer than women who did not take hormones. In 1997, three researchers reviewed the benefits of HRT for women after menopause and concluded that by reducing the risks of serious diseases, "HRT should increase life expectancy for nearly all postmenopausal women by up to 3 years."[2]

So it is no wonder that in her 1995 book *A New Prescription for Women's Health: Getting the Best Medical Care in a Man's World*, Bernadine Healy, a cardiologist and the first female director of the National Institutes of Health (NIH), observed that many of the major risks that women face as they age — heart disease, stroke, osteoporosis, and Alzheimer's disease — "are or may well be reduced by hormone replacement therapy." As a result of those data, she said, when she hit menopause, she planned to begin HRT "without a blink." The benefits are remarkable, she wrote, not only for reducing the risk of specific diseases but also for improving a woman's "total health" and quality of life, giving a woman, in effect, a "second prime."[3] She added: "A decision not to consider hormone replacement is a health decision, too, just as is the decision not to take a flu shot or get a hepatitis vaccination. As I see it, women have a competitive health and survival edge before menopause. Women during their childbearing years are protected against many problems that affect men. I see no reason to relinquish that advantage after menopause — not if I can help it."

*   *   *

And that's where matters stood until July 8, 2002, when the National Institutes of Health issued a press release that immediately got the attention of every physician, every woman in menopause, and every medical journalist around the world: "The National Heart, Lung, and Blood Institute of the NIH has stopped early the Women's Health Initiative, a major clinical trial of the risks and benefits of combined oestrogen and progestin in healthy menopausal women due to an increased risk of invasive breast cancer." The *Journal of the American Medical Association* (JAMA), in advance of publishing the paper, added in its own press release that the WHI study was stopped not only because of increased breast cancer risk, but also because of increased risks of coronary heart disease, stroke, and pulmonary embolisms.[4]

These press releases generated an avalanche of panic-inducing headlines: "HRT Linked to Breast Cancer," announced the BBC. "Hormone Replacement Study a Shock to the Medical System," said the *New York Times*. The article quoted Wulf Utian, an obstetrician-gynecologist who was also executive director of the North American Menopause Society: "This is the biggest bombshell that ever hit in my 30-something years in the menopause area."

It certainly was. The WHI was and is the largest prospective study in which women were randomized to take either hormones or a placebo and then followed over time. Its increasing cost now totals more than one billion dollars; its investigators are leading physicians, statisticians, and epidemiologists across the country; and ongoing analyses of its findings continue to be published in medicine's most prestigious journals. No wonder the announcement caused a panic among the millions of women taking hormones. Already frightened of breast cancer, hundreds of thousands went off hormone replacement immediately; the prescription rate for HRT quickly fell by up to 70 percent[5] and it remains low to this day. Most of these women's physicians supported this decision, and many medical centers rely on the WHI's conclusions and advise women not to take HRT at all or to take it only briefly.

Confusion trailed panic; *Newsweek* summed it up in a long article headlined "What's a Woman to Do?" Should women who have menopausal symptoms deny themselves the benefits of HRT, in the short term or over many years, to avoid increasing the risk of breast cancer and cardiovascular disease? One researcher described the WHI's "melodramatic presentation of its results" as being guaranteed to generate "shock, terror and controversy" in the media. It set the tone for all early reporting about the study and created massive confusion about HRT.[6]

Unfortunately, my medical colleagues and I had to wait eight days before the WHI's official report was published in *JAMA*. "Publication by press conference" is always suspicious, because reporters, scientists, and physicians can't immediately examine the researchers' claims. The frightening findings make headlines and the incorrect conclusions circulate around the world before the truth gets out of bed. When I was finally able to read the actual study, I could not believe my eyes. None of the claims about breast cancer were statistically or medically strong (or *significant*, in research language). Breast cancer had not even been the WHI's primary focus; its goal was to study heart disease in women long *past* menopause.

I watched with growing puzzlement and irritation as the drumbeat of bad news from the WHI continued over the years: Oestrogen doesn't improve the quality of life for women in menopause, researchers said in 2003.[7] (Martha was highly amused by that one.) Others claimed that it increased the risk of ovarian cancer and of death from lung cancer, shortened women's lives, and hastened cognitive decline and dementia. Scary stories emerged in the news every couple of years, like the flu, and then faded away.

Now, I am trained as a scientist. I'm willing—indeed, I am *obligated*—to examine studies that would make me reassess my beliefs and change how I practice medicine. Thus, with each headline and each new round of fearmongering, I dove headfirst into a close examination of the WHI's data and their researchers' analyses. The more I read, the angrier I became. Many of those claims were exaggerated, some were misleading, and some were just plain wrong. I cannot overstate how shocking this realization was. The Women's Health Initiative—a randomized, double-blind study, the gold standard of empirical research, funded by the National Institutes of Health—and its findings couldn't be trusted? Exactly right, and by the time you finish this book, you will see why.

No wonder I began getting letters like this one, from a former patient who had moved to another city:

Dear Dr. Bluming:

Today I had an appointment with Dr. L to renew my prescription for the hormones I have been taking. She quickly told me to find another doctor as she could not and would not prescribe HRT. In order for someone to be given hormones, she said, the patient would have to be no older than 62 or so (I am much older) and have hot flashes — which I do not have because I am on hormones. She would not continue to treat me if I insisted on remaining on hormones. These medicines have helped me a great deal and provided me with a life, instead of days of sitting on the sofa or in bed unable to move or think. What do I do? Who can I see? Are there other drugs I can take in their place? How can I find a doctor to support me and track what is needed?

As I read my patient's letter, I wondered how her oncologist had become so adamantly opposed to hormone replacement therapy that she was unable to recognize its benefits in the woman sitting in front of her, who had been on HRT for more than twenty years.

Carol's Story:

Avrum and I have been close friends for many years. We met when Avrum saved my sister-in-law's life with a successful intervention for a rare blood disorder caused by a stroke medication. We discovered a mutual passion for following the data wherever it led and a shared commitment to debunking pseudoscience and fad therapies, Av in medicine, I in psychology. The story of HRT—a therapy praised by some researchers and women's health activists, condemned by others—was fascinating in its own right but it also perfectly combined two of my lifelong interests: gender biases in health care and cognitive biases in research.

One afternoon shortly after the Women's Health Initiative's famous press conference in 2002, I decided to attend Avrum's talk about HRT at his weekly continuing medical education seminar. I went mostly out of friendship; I didn't have a strong opinion about hormone replacement one way or the other, and I had sailed through menopause with nary a symptom. In my 1992 book *The Mismeasure of Woman*, I included a chapter on hormone replacement, a therapy I didn't wholly oppose but didn't wholly endorse either. In those years, I shared the view of many feminists (generally those who, like me, were premenopausal) that the idea of hormone "replacement" was itself problematic, implying that this normal change of life created deficiencies and was a pathology to be medically corrected and not simply, well, a normal change of life.

And then I watched, riveted, as Avrum methodically dismantled the arguments that HRT was a serious risk factor in breast cancer. He presented a table of breast cancer risks, which you will see in chapter 1, that soon had his audience laughing out loud. At the least risky end was taking HRT, the WHI's "finding" that had caused such concern. Riskier factors included eating one additional serving of French fries per week during preschool years, eating grapefruit, working night shifts, and being a Scandinavian airline flight attendant.

I was jolted out of my seat. I realized that Avrum was doing in medicine what I loved doing in psychology: presenting evidence that contradicted received wisdom and dealing with people's exasperating reaction to such evidence. (A hint: They rarely say "Thank you.") I was therefore not surprised when Av told me how much trouble he was having in trying to persuade his colleagues that they might be wrong about the dangers of HRT and the reliability of the Women's Health Initiative. We collaborated on three articles for medical journals (the *Cancer Journal* and *Climacteric*[8]) and in 2022, the *Cancer Journal* invited him to be guest editor of a special issue on oestrogen.

But for both of us, the most important audience for this information is women; after all, it's their lives and their health that is at stake. And so we decided to write this book, directed to general readers but with all the supporting research a physician would want to judge our arguments. In chapter 1 we consider the effects of hormone replacement therapy on menopausal symptoms, which are so varied that many women and their doctors have no idea that their common cause is oestrogen depletion. In the next two chapters we address women's deep fear of breast cancer and the widespread assumption that oestrogen is carcinogenic: *Does* oestrogen cause breast cancer? And can breast cancer survivors take oestrogen? Chapters 4, 5, and 6 review oestrogen's benefits in reducing women's risks of heart disease, osteoporosis, diabetes, colon cancer, and dementia, and increasing their longevity. Chapter 7 examines women's concerns about progesterone and the birth control pill. The final chapter reviews the issues and take-home lessons in the case for HRT.

*   *   *

We are well aware that many women's health activists assume that all advocates for oestrogen are in the pocket of Big Pharma and thus cannot be trusted. We therefore want to make it clear that neither of us has been paid anything by Wyeth (purchased by Pfizer in 2009) or any other drug company. Both of us are appalled by Wyeth's stranglehold on the patent for Premarin—among the most popular versions of oestrogen—and the outrageously high cost to women who greatly benefit from it. I have long been an outspoken critic of the pharmaceutical industry, and Avrum has never met with drug reps in his office, let alone accepted dinners, pens, speaking offers, writing assignments, pizzas, or any other bribe or inducement in exchange for writing a particular prescription.[9]

Oestrogen Matters Update, 2024

In the years since this book was first published in 2018, women are becoming more vocal about menopause. Cohorts of women do this, of course, every time they reach the "change." What is different now is the emergence of a generation of women who are not passive about taking charge of their lives and health, and who do not regard menopause as a shame or a scandal. What is different now is that women are angry that physicians are taught almost nothing about menopause in medical school, have no idea of the diverse symptoms of menopause and perimenopause, and overlook or trivialize women's specific menopausal complaints and experiences. What is different now is the emergence of an exploding menopause market to address and monetize their concerns; these businesses sell products and services (such as expensive "menopause retreats" at spas and resorts) as well as advice. As the podcast *The Daily* put it in an episode on July 28, 2023, "Menopause is having a moment." That's a multibillion-dollar moment, thank you; websites, books, specialists, concierge services, and potions and placebos for treatment are proliferating. Silence about menopause has been replaced by a cacophony of voices. How should a woman find her way through them?

For us, it meant that the "moment" was right to update this book, reporting new findings of relevance to women who, with their physicians, are deciding whether hormone therapy is right for them. Throughout, we bring readers up to date on the WHI. With nary a press conference or a "good news about hormone therapy!" headline to inform them, the public is largely unaware that the WHI has walked back virtually all of its early alarmist findings. The FDA continues to require an ominous black box on every oestrogen product, warning of "cardiovascular disease, probable dementia, and breast cancer." And yet the WHI investigators now say that oestrogen does *not* increase deaths from heart disease and cancer. On the contrary, it increases longevity, most notably when begun within ten years of the last menstrual period. HRT is the best preventive for osteoporotic hip fractures. It is safe and effective when applied vaginally for local symptoms. And, in the most striking about-face from their 2003 headlines that HRT "did not have a clinically meaningful effect on health-related quality of life" for women in menopause, they stated in 2019 and again in 2021 that "hormone therapy is the most effective treatment for managing menopausal vasomotor symptoms" and thereby improving women's quality of life.[10] How many women know this? That's the problem.

As for women who avoid oestrogen because of their deep-seated fears of breast cancer, we updated these two crucial chapters and show how the belief that oestrogen causes breast cancer has blinded otherwise reputable, serious investigators to what their own data reveals. In 2020, for example, the WHI investigators reported a decreased incidence of breast cancer among women randomized to oestrogen after 19 years of follow-up.[11] This is crucial information for women who have had hysterectomies and therefore would take oestrogen on its own. It's the combination of oestrogen and progesterone (HRT), the WHI still maintains, that raises the risk.[12] But as we will show in chapter 2, that finding was due to a statistical misinterpretation: The women on HRT did not have an *increased* risk; the control group had a *reduced* risk, because many of the women in that group had been on oestrogen before the study. When they were removed from analysis, the supposed increased risk of HRT vanished.[13] Because this news is of major importance, we provide a deep dive into the statistical thickets to show what re-analyses of the WHI's one remaining argument against HRT have revealed.

In *Monty Python and the Holy Grail,* the Black Knight loses first his left arm to King Arthur's sword, then his right arm, and then both legs. Nonetheless, the Black Knight will not admit defeat: "'Tis but a scratch," he says. The WHI has done its damnedest to kill HRT, ignoring the well-grounded criticisms of its methods and findings as if they were scratches. We are pleased to be part of a new generation of health activists, ob-gyns, and medical researchers who are working hard to lay the Black Knight to rest.

Why does it matter? In the years since this book first appeared, hundreds of women—from the United States, United Kingdom, Poland, Portugal, Brazil, Thailand, Bangladesh, and everywhere in between—have written to Avrum, and in this revision we include some of their voices and questions. They tell him over and over that their doctors do not listen to them, do not hear their stories, and refuse to prescribe oestrogen, even when they had safely been taking it for many years to alleviate their suffering. Their doctors might not listen, but we have.

1

The "Change of Life" and the Quality of Life

When Oprah Winfrey was 46 years old, she developed attacks of severe heart palpitations. She saw at least five cardiologists, each of whom assured her that her heart was fine, but none of them could tell her what was causing the palpitations. She was frustrated, especially because, as she observed to her legions of fans in her magazine, no physician would want to misdiagnose her since she was, in fact, Oprah Winfrey. She remained worried and annoyed by the palpitations until her trainer suggested that they could be a sign of early menopause.[1] "Of course it's not menopause!" she said. "I'm still having my periods. Regular as rain!" But then she came upon a popular book, *The Wisdom of Menopause* by Dr. Christiane Northrup, that listed palpitations as a common symptom of menopause.

Heart palpitations certainly get a woman's attention, but other symptoms that are also signs of menopause usually do not, symptoms such as severe dryness of the eyes and mouth, which many women develop even when they are still having regular periods, or joint and muscle aches and pains. The list of symptoms associated with menopause includes other surprises as well as the familiar ones.

Hot flushes (the popular but less accurate term is hot *flashes*)
Night sweats
Difficulty sleeping
Insomnia
Difficulty concentrating
Decreasing recent memory
Decreasing energy reserve
Bladder/urinary discomfort
More frequent urinary tract infections
Vaginal dryness
Vaginal discharge
Vaginal bleeding
Loss of sexual desire
Painful sexual intercourse
Depression/sadness
Anxiety
Tension/nervousness
Mood swings
Headaches
Bloating
Swelling of hands or feet
Breast tenderness

Aching joints
Thinning hair
Palpitations (racing or irregular heartbeat)
Chest pain with exertion
Dry mouth (diminished saliva)
Weight gain around the abdomen

That last entry is, of course, the lament of many women confronted with the dilemma of "Do I accept this change in waist size and get new clothes? Or do I wage war against the forces of biology and eat nothing but protein and work out three times a day?" People joke about "middle-aged spread" and usually attribute it to sloth, fast food, and too much sugar, but for women, menopause is also a major contributor. "I weigh the same as I always did," one of Av's patients grumbled, "but my fat cells seem to have redistributed themselves and reconvened in my belly."

The symptoms of menopause often begin in the years before periods stop completely (known as perimenopause) and can last for years afterward. But many women do not mention them to their doctors at all, let alone in any detail, sometimes because of shame or embarrassment, but often because, like Oprah Winfrey, they don't associate the problem with menopause. Heart palpitations send many women to cardiologists; aching muscles and joints send them to rheumatologists; insomnia sends them to sleep-disorder clinics; and depression sends them to psychotherapists or psychiatrists. One 50-year-old woman we spoke to said, "I had suffered from insomnia for years, attributing it to work stresses and the kids. But once I started HRT, I slept soundly through the night for the first time in four years. The work is still stressful and the kids are still kids, but I sleep." Another said that when she entered menopause in her early fifties, she had none of the concerns her friends did—no hot flushes, no sleepless nights, no headaches—and so she didn't consider taking hormones. "Then, one night," she said, "I dreamed that I was happy—really happy—and when I awoke I realized I had not felt that joyful in too long. I didn't know that one symptom of menopause is depression. I called my doctor and began HRT right away, and I became my cheerful self again. I took it for years but stopped because she advised me to, after the WHI reports. I am still seething that I quit."

Echoing the complaints and concerns of many women in Av's practice, one psychotherapist wrote to us with her own observations:

> Every day in my practice I work with women who—either through their doctors' discouragement or due to their own fears and misinformation—have not taken oestrogen and experienced its benefits. I see major depression and generalized anxiety disorder, ruined sexual and emotional connection with spouses, disintegrating marriages and fractured families as a result. Of course, the depletion of oestrogen in menopause is not the single cause of these problems, but I'm certain it plays a predominant role in the abrupt loss of these women's (and their families') quality of life after menopause.

Oh, it does. In *The Madwoman in the Volvo: My Year of Raging Hormones,* Sandra Tsing Loh's hilarious account of her midlife crisis induced by menopause, the author describes the miseries of being "oestrogen-deprived," many of which are funny (at least afterward, and at least when described by a professional humorist).

There she is, pulling off the road to sob—"producing heaves of seawater like Jonah's whale"—about the death of her children's hamster: "I am a forty-nine-year-old woman sitting in her filthy Volvo parked under a tree on a Tuesday afternoon wailing about a hamster. Just how low are we setting the bar here?" (Though, she adds, it was an adorable hamster with a sunny disposition.) Her good friend Ann, hearing the story, gently suggests Loh might be entering menopause. But the fanatical regimen that Ann has adopted to deal with her depression and rage attacks—"a cocktail of antidepressants, bioidenticals, walks, facials, massages, dark chocolate, and practically throwing salt over her shoulder"—does not help Loh. Eventually, Loh finds salvation and sanity in putting topical oestrogen cream on her wrists.[2]

Individual experiences are illuminating but they are not scientific evidence; for one thing, people are often famously incorrect about the causes of their physical and emotional concerns. For example, starting in their fifties, both sexes tend to gain weight. Many women are so hyperalert to their weight that they latch onto any culprit they can blame, but at least the ones who aren't taking hormones can rule out HRT. "There is a general belief among women and even some doctors that menopause hormones contribute to weight gain," wrote Tara Parker-Pope in *The Hormone Decision*. "The scientific data simply do not support this."[3] In a large, yearlong study that compared menopausal women on hormones with those who were on a placebo, most of the women gained some weight—but the hormone group gained less than the placebo group. And in the Women's Health Initiative (WHI), a higher proportion of those on HRT *lost* weight compared to the women on placebo.[4]

Everyone knows that depression, anxiety, marital unhappiness, and sexual problems occur for many different reasons — physiological, psychological, and fighting with one's partner. But in this chapter, we will argue that the drop in oestrogen is an underrecognized cause of the wide array of symptoms that emerge during menopause. We will consider the evidence showing why oestrogen remains the most effective treatment for these symptoms, and we will evaluate the claims that bioidentical products or alternative therapies are just as effective as oestrogen without the alleged risks. But first we want to acknowledge the historical, cultural, and political context of this contentious issue.

OESTROGEN: THE JEKYLL AND HYDE OF TREATMENTS

Over its long history, oestrogen has been seen as everything from a cure-all for any and every female complaint to a dangerous, even disastrous drug; from a kindly Dr. Jekyll to a fiendish Mr. Hyde; from the solution to the problem. "The story of oestrogen," Elizabeth Siegel Watkins wrote in *The Estrogen Elixir,* her fascinating history of HRT in America, "is woven from several strands: blind faith in the ability of science and technology to solve a broad range of health and social problems, social and cultural stigmatization of aging, shifting meanings and interpretations of femininity and female identity, and the pitfalls of medical hubris in the twentieth century."[5] Women wanting to make decisions about hormone replacement therapy struggle to untangle those strands. Is taking HRT antifeminist or profeminist? Why is *replacement* a bad word when it refers to menopause hormones but not a bad word when it refers to, say, replacing thyroid hormones if the thyroid gland is removed? (And given that, after menopause, oestrogen levels in many women drop to as low as 1 percent of what they were before menopause, *replacement* seems precisely the right word.[6]) Does HRT medicalize a problem that would be better treated with psychotherapy or a new job? Is it healthier to tough it out and suffer in silence or try hormones?

The 1970s, with the birth of the modern feminist movement, saw a sharp split emerge among feminists on the subject of oestrogen. The decade was off to a roaring start with *Our Bodies, Ourselves,* a book that was greeted with well-deserved fanfare in 1971; it urged women to learn about their bodies, health, and sexuality and take control of their own medical care. In 1977, two popular books anchored the feminist anti-oestrogen position: Rosetta Reitz's *Menopause: A Positive Approach* and Barbara and Gideon Seaman's *Women and the Crisis in Sex Hormones.* As Watkins wrote, "These two books reflected the contemporary critical stance against the organized medical profession and the pharmaceutical industry and the concurrent fascination with so-called natural approaches to health care."[7] Those natural approaches, still recommended, were exercise, calcium, "good nutrition" (however it was defined that year), and, for Reitz, perhaps telling us more about herself than the general population, having regular sex and healthy relationships. Both of these successful books regarded hormone therapy of any kind as either unnecessary or harmful. But their main strengths lay in their clarion call to women to resist the paternalism of the establishment and reject the insulting language of menopause as being a "deficiency disease" and the pervasive, sexist notion that once past menopause, women were, literally and figuratively, washed up.

Yet the very success of feminism was sending more women into science, research, and medicine. In the same year that Reitz and the Seamans published their books, Lila Nachtigall, an obstetrician-gynecologist at NYU who at the time was halfway through her own 22-year research study, produced *The Lila Nachtigall Report*. The book urged women to educate themselves, and it provided comprehensive information about menopause and the therapeutic benefits of oestrogen. Nachtigall entered medical school in 1956, one of four women in her class, and has worked as an advocate for women ever since. But in the newly exuberant feminism of the 1970s, Watkins observed, "*The Lila Nachtigall Report* didn't stand a chance. Written by a doctor who was promoting the use of a drug that was at the nadir of its popularity, castigated by scientists and feminists alike, the book was out of step with the times."[8] Nine years later, in 1986, when Nachtigall wrote *Estrogen: The Facts Can Change Your Life*, the climate had changed. The benefits of oestrogen—in preventing osteoporosis (Nachtigall's specialty) and promoting heart health—were repeatedly demonstrated. Until, of course, the Women's Health Initiative set that pendulum swinging back again.

Many feminists and health activists continue to oppose HRT for social and political reasons as well as health concerns. After the WHI's press release in 2002, Cynthia Pearson, then executive director of the National Women's Health Network, told Gina Kolata of the *New York Times* how pleased she was that the WHI had validated her opposition to HRT. The advocacy of HRT, she told Kolata, was "sexist and ageist, with its message that women should: Stay healthy. Stay sexually vital. Be less of a pain to your husband."[9]

Sexist and ageist, really? At a conference devoted to the treatment of oestrogen-deficiency symptoms, Nachtigall noted: "Among 2,000 postmenopausal women in a given year, 20 will develop heart disease, 11 bone loss, 6 breast cancer, and 3 endometrial cancer, but nearly 100 percent will develop urogenital atrophy. Urogenital atrophy is not the first sign of menopause, but rather occurs gradually after the onset of the climacteric."[10] The symptoms include vaginal itching, urinary burning, urinary frequency, more frequent urinary infections, and painful sexual intercourse. During menopause, tissues that rely on oestrogen become thin and lose elasticity, which is why urogenital atrophy, if left untreated, will persist and worsen as a woman ages. *Urogenital atrophy* has at least replaced the obnoxious and misleading term *vaginal atrophy*. *Atrophy* simply refers to a loss or thinning of tissue, and urogenital atrophy involves the bladder and other organs as well as the vagina and vulva.

We are fully aware of the many women, and men, whose attitude toward sex in their later years is "free at last"; we do not wish to imply that everyone wants, or should want, to be sexually active. Some will find greater sensual pleasures in golf, opera, or tango dancing. But we think it is just as misguided to assume that most women in their middle and late years do *not* want to be sexually active. To see the bias, reread that list of symptoms at the start of this chapter, omitting breast tenderness and vaginal discomfort, as if it applied to men. How would men respond to being told, "Buck up, guys! It's normal aging! Don't worry about those chest pains and bloating and headaches, the sleepless nights and memory lapses! No interest in sex anymore? Painful intercourse? Hey, you're over 50; you've had enough sex already. Oh, your wife still enjoys sex? Too bad; be less of a pain to her about it. Besides, those symptoms will last only a few years, though more than half of you men will still have those symptoms for another decade or more, and some of you will have painful intercourse from now on. A lubricant will help if you want sex, but it won't help you want sex."

It would be hard to imagine most men accepting that message.

Of course, we know what Pearson meant by "ageist"—the ubiquitous cultural message that old is bad, young is good, and all of us, men and women alike, should fight signs of age with every weapon at hand. The non-ageist view held by many feminists is that the symptoms of menopause are as normal a part of life as menarche and therefore something to be tolerated, while repeating the mantra of King Solomon: "This too shall pass." If symptoms are severe, they can be treated with alternatives to medication. In this view, menopause can be dealt with in the same way that people deal with any other sign of age, such as gray hair or wrinkles: try some over-the-counter aids or do nothing. A friend of ours, a college professor, hated having hot flushes and the resultant profusion of sweat that left her drenched, but she treated it all matter-of-factly, once telling her class: "This is what hot flashes look like. I'm not about to faint or die. Now hand in your papers."

Moreover, we share Pearson's and other consumer advocates' criticism of Big Pharma's unregulated ability to advertise directly to consumers, generate new medications by barely changing a molecule in older, effective ones, and expand markets for medications where none are needed. We too are sympathetic to the Less Is More movement, which is trying to educate the public so they will avoid unnecessary medications and diagnostic tests. We too condemn "disease-mongering," the arbitrary creation of new diseases, usually done by extending the borders of real physical conditions to include "pre-" conditions that do not and may never need medication. (As we will discuss in chapter 5, *osteopenia,* allegedly a precursor of osteoporosis, is one such manufactured term, propelled to its status, as one medical historian wrote, "by aggressive marketing and vested interests."[11])

We can't deny that oestrogen too has had aggressive marketing and vested interests behind it. In 1942, researchers developed methods to extract large quantities of oestrogen from the urine of pregnant mares, and Ayerst Laboratories produced the first oestrogen tablets, which they called Premarin (from *preg*nant *mares'* ur*ine*). Ayerst began to market Premarin in the 1950s as a treatment for menopausal symptoms, a campaign greatly enhanced by *Feminine Forever* (1966), a hyperventilating bestseller written by New York gynecologist Robert Wilson.[12] The book promised youth, beauty, and a full sex life for menopausal women through the use of oestrogen. Wilson's son Ronald later told reporter Gina Kolata at the *New York Times* that Ayerst had paid all the expenses involved in writing the book and financed his father's organization, the Wilson Research Foundation.[13]

In the years following that book's publication, many physicians handed out hormones readily and pressured their patients to take them and not ask pesky questions. It's not a surprise that these doctors were often arrogant and sexist, given that menopause was described in their textbooks as a "deficiency disease" or "ovarian failure."[14] And it's no surprise that many feminists were skeptical of HRT's benefits; it was hard to separate the question of hormones from the condescension of the (mostly) men prescribing them. Carol's mother, Dorie, loved telling the story of what happened when her gynecologist asked when she had had her last period.

"Hmm," she'd said, reflecting. "It's been about a year, come to think of it."

"Are you having hot flashes, sleeplessness, aches, and pains?" he asked.

"No," she said, "though I did have a chill in a movie theater once."

"Here," he said, not listening, "have this prescription filled; it will help."

Years have gone by since that conversation, and the needle of oestrogen advice has moved from pro to con. Today, we are convinced that having that prescription filled *will* often help, after all.

MENOPAUSE AND BEYOND

Menopause — the cessation of fertility in females who live many years afterward — is something of an evolutionary mystery. As neuroscientist Lisa Mosconi writes in *The Menopause Brain*, the only animal species known to outlive their fertility are "certain whales, some Asian elephants, possibly some giraffes, and one insect, the Japanese aphid."[15] In 2023, researchers found that menopause occurs in our nearest relative, the chimpanzee. In a group of 185 female chimps in Uganda, fertility began to decline after age 30 (as it does in other chimp groups and humans), and menopause, the end of fertility, occurred around age 50. Yet many of the chimps lived long past 50, with the same declining levels of oestrogens and progestins seen in human women.[16]

Thus, the once-common belief that menopause is an evolutionary fluke is yielding to the grandmother hypothesis, the view that it is an evolutionary adaptation. The grandmother hypothesis holds that in ancient times, human infants and children were more likely to survive if their grandmothers were around to care for them and were not in sexual competition with their daughters for partners and resources.[17] The evolutionary explanation for chimp menopause is somewhat different, because older chimp females live apart from their daughters and migrate to a new group. Because of menopause, they do not compete with younger fertile females and pose no competitive threat. But whatever the evolutionary reason for menopause, due to the extraordinary advances in health and sanitation in the past century, women live an average of three decades after menopause, making the issue of improving their health and their quality of life more pressing.

Some women have virtually no symptoms during menopause; like Carol and her mother, their periods just stop, and that's that. But they are a minority. According to the Study of Women's Health Across the Nation (SWAN), a multiracial/multiethnic study that ran from 1996 to 2013 and followed more than 3,000 women as they entered menopause, about 80 percent of women experience some symptoms, and for half of them, those symptoms last for years. The median duration of hot flushes and other vasomotor symptoms among these women was 7.4 years; it was longer (10 years) for Black women and upwards of 12 years for women whose symptoms began during perimenopause.[18] Black and Latina women also enter perimenopause much sooner on average, sometimes even in their thirties, so their symptoms start much earlier and can be more severe. Needless to say—but we will say it—many doctors are unaware of this important information or of their biases toward minority women, who are finally speaking out about their experiences and needs.[19]

The Women's Health Initiative did not even want to grant that HRT might help alleviate these unpleasant symptoms. The WHI reported in 2003 that oestrogen did not have a "clinically meaningful effect on health-related quality of life," even among women who had taken it for three years.[20] When Av's wife, Martha, read this news, she laughed out loud. She had been pushed into menopause at the age of 46 as a result of chemotherapy and almost immediately developed hot flushes, night sweats, severe bladder pain, and difficulty sleeping. Martha started oestrogen, and within days, her symptoms diminished, then disappeared. It usually takes less than a week for most symptomatic menopausal women to feel better after beginning HRT; how in the world did the WHI get such an anomalous result?

When their study began, the WHI researchers were not interested in the effect of hormones on menopausal symptoms; they were investigating the hormones' effects on the big problems, primarily heart disease and, secondarily, breast cancer and cognitive impairment. Then why did they publish an article on the menopausal symptoms they had not set out to study? We don't know, but it feels to us that they were reluctant to admit that HRT was beneficial to women for *anything*.

We say this because the WHI researchers wrote that they explicitly discouraged women who reported having "moderate or severe" menopausal symptoms from participating. As a result, women who had moderate or severe symptoms made up only 13 percent of the study participants. (Moreover, their median age was 63, so most of the symptoms they might have had at the onset of menopause and for the subsequent decade had passed.) However, among those 13 percent with symptoms, more than three-fourths randomized to take HRT rather than placebo reported substantial relief—just as every other study has found. The rest of the sample, the women who had had either no symptoms or minimal symptoms, reported no relief of symptoms. Let's repeat that: *The women who didn't have symptoms reported that oestrogen did not relieve the symptoms they didn't have.* And that is how the WHI got its "finding" that HRT did not have a "clinically meaningful effect on health-related quality of life"[21]—by focusing on the 87 percent who had had no symptoms at the outset and were way past menopause in any case. The authors themselves noted that their data "may not be applicable to [women with moderate to severe symptoms], because women who believed they needed hormone therapy were unlikely to agree to undergo randomization."

We are not making this up.

Another way the WHI could claim that HRT did not improve quality of life was in how the investigators measured quality of life. They didn't offer participants a list of specific symptoms and ask them to assess the severity of each one, ranging from "not at all troubling" to "tolerable" to "unbearable" and note whether and how each symptom was affecting their lives. Instead, they relied on vague assessments, asking participants to rate their well-being, mood, ways of coping, and general health. When people are asked for global evaluations like these, they typically respond as you probably do when an acquaintance asks you how you are. You most likely say, "Oh, I'm fine. All good." You don't mention the sweats, sleeplessness, palpitations, and problems with your partner, boss, kids, and noisy neighbors. (Similarly, on national opinion polls, when people are asked how happy they are overall, about two-thirds say "very happy." Ask them about particular aspects of their lives and you'll get the truth: "My shoulder pain has finally gone away but I'm super-stressed by my boss and ready to send my sullen teenager to boot camp.") Global assessments, in short, play off women's tendency to cope and not complain about particular symptoms that are interfering with work or family life.

But even the WHI could not overturn the consensus that oestrogen is the most effective treatment for the symptoms that Martha had and millions of other women have, eliminating or reducing them in the great majority of women who take HRT or oestrogen only. "To this day," wrote Elizabeth Watkins in 2007, "oestrogen remains the single most effective remedy for the hot flashes of menopause, and few critics dispute its value as a temporary treatment."[22] Multiple randomized trials reviewed by oncologist Heidi Nelson of the Mayo Clinic found that oestrogen generally reduces the frequency of hot flushes by more than 75 percent.[23]

The WISDOM study, an acronym for the Women's International Study of Long-Duration Oestrogen After the Menopause, was a randomized, placebo-controlled trial of 3,721 postmenopausal women in Australia, New Zealand, and the United Kingdom. The women ranged in age from 50 to 69 and were randomly assigned to take HRT or placebo. Compared to the women given the placebo, women on HRT experienced improved sleep, reduced hot flushes and night sweats, fewer aching joints and muscles, less vaginal dryness, and improved sexual functioning.[24] The researchers particularly emphasized the benefits of HRT on improving sleep and reducing insomnia, given that inadequate sleep is "associated with an increased risk of illnesses such as obesity, diabetes, hypertension, and cardiovascular disease. Reducing sleep deprivation might therefore have considerable health benefits."

Further, because many menopausal women report joint and muscle pain and increased arthritic symptoms — as we said, that's another set of symptoms not popularly associated with menopause — the WISDOM researchers highlighted their finding that women reported lower levels of bodily pain after a year on HRT. Indeed, they cited the WHI, which had (quietly) gotten the same result: "A follow-up study with participants in the Women's Health Initiative that looked at joint symptoms showed a higher prevalence of pain or stiffness in those women who stopped taking combined HRT compared with placebo."[25] Research on animals, they added, suggested that oestrogen also "has an anaesthetic role and might prevent cartilage erosion such as occurs in osteoarthritis."[26]

Although the WISDOM study found no alleviation of symptoms of depression among the participants, two randomized trials of oestrogen therapy reported remarkable success. Women suffering from depressive episodes received four to twelve weeks of oestrogen or placebo. Those in the oestrogen group had a 60 to 75 percent improvement versus a 20 to 30 percent improvement for women given placebo.[27] That oestrogen was so much better than antidepressants, and without the side effects antidepressants often have,[28] should have been big news. Katie Taylor, a British woman, was her own control group in experiencing the difference between antidepressants and HRT:

A few years ago, I was 43, and had just returned to work after a long break bringing up my four children. I loved my life, but was feeling exhausted, teary and down, for no obvious reason. My GP [general practitioner] diagnosed depression and prescribed anti-depressants. This, it turned out, was a misdiagnosis. After six months, I felt worse. I had "brain fog," couldn't think clearly at work, cried at the most inconvenient moments, had hot flushes and didn't want to leave the house.... The anti-depressant turned me into a zombie, I felt nothing—it just wasn't right. I feared it was the pressure of combining home life with a demanding job.... I talked to my GP again and she agreed I should stop working and focus on my own health and looking after my family.[29]

That "stop working" was more bad advice, and it is advice that most women can't afford to take anyway. Fortunately for Katie Taylor, she was the daughter of Michael Baum, one of England's preeminent cancer researchers, and he suggested that, young as she was, she might be in menopause. And that was the right diagnosis; she was indeed. She began HRT, got off the antidepressant, "got the old Katie back" with her former cheerfulness and energy, and even started an online support group to provide information for women going through menopause.

Many gynecologists and oncologists still struggle to reconcile their conviction that oestrogen is dangerous and doesn't improve quality of life with the clear evidence of its benefits. They have come up with a curious compromise: it is safe for *some* women with severe symptoms to take hormones if they do it for the briefest time and in the smallest dose possible. This advice represents a compromise between "It's dangerous; don't take it at all" and "It's safe; take it as long as you like." Of course, if physicians really believe that oestrogen is carcinogenic, they shouldn't advise taking it at all; that is like saying, "Smoke a half a pack of cigarettes a day, but only for a year, and you'll sleep better."

This is the bottom line: *There is no scientific basis for the admonition to take as low a dose of postmenopausal hormones for as short a period as possible.* Guidelines from the American College of Obstetrics and Gynecology state that "because some women age 65 or more might still need HRT for vasomotor symptoms, HRT should not be routinely discontinued at age 65, but, as in younger women, should be individualized."[30] The North American Menopause Society concurs: "The concept of 'lowest dose for the shortest time' may be inadequate or even harmful for some women...there are no data to support routine discontinuation [of HRT] in women age 65 years."[31]

In 2012, ten years after their original scare stories, the WHI researchers admitted that oestrogen does, in fact, significantly reduce vasomotor symptoms such as lightheadedness, dizziness, and hot flushes, symptoms that recur as soon as women stop taking oestrogen.[32] One of the principal investigators, JoAnn Manson, allowed that women could now safely take HRT without fear that it would cause early death: "This is good news for women," she told the *Times* (UK). "This fundamentally provides reassurance for women during the menopause who are seeking hormone therapy to manage bothersome and disturbing symptoms such as hot flushes and night sweats."[33] (The *Times* offered a bold headline yet to be seen in American papers: "Women Told Hormone Replacement Therapy Does Not Lead to Early Death.") Three years later, in 2015, Manson and her colleague Gloria Richard-Davis went further. In "Research Overturns Dogma," a commentary on that large-scale SWAN study, they commended the researchers for overturning "the dogma that [vasomotor symptoms] have a short duration, minimally affect women's health or quality of life and can be readily addressed by short-term approaches."[34]

They praised the overturning of the dogma that they themselves created? While we regret that Manson and colleagues originally promoted the inappropriately alarmist interpretations of the WHI findings, not even recognizing HRT's benefits on menopausal symptoms, we are pleased that they have been able to change their minds — a little. "There was a lot of fear," Manson told the *Times*, not quite admitting that it was primarily the WHI that generated that fear.

We are also pleased that, by 2021, Manson and her associates concurred that "for the vast majority of symptomatic women, the benefits of HRT outweigh the risks. It is imperative that the choice of treatment be individualized and that patients share in the decision making."[35]

We could not agree more, which is why we are sorry to see that the WHI investigators are still to-ing and fro-ing on the matter of HRT's risks versus benefits. In that 2021 paper, they reported that after 13 years of follow-up, HRT did *not* increase the risk of venous thromboembolism or stroke. But in 2023, they said that it *did* increase the risk of thromboembolism and stroke and so, they concluded, "vasomotor symptoms should only be treated if they are bothersome." They referred to these symptoms, which can disrupt sleep for years and impair quality of life, as merely "bothersome"? Wasn't that the dogma they were glad had been overturned? And, disagreeing with the guidelines from the American College of Obstetrics and Gynecology and the North American Menopause Society, they maintained that "clinicians should prescribe the lowest effective dose of hormone therapy for the shortest duration consistent with the patient's needs, with periodic reevaluation of the need for continued hormone therapy to control symptoms."[36]

If leading WHI investigators can't decide whether the benefits of HRT outweigh the risks, or the risks outweigh the benefits, and resort to that unsatisfying recommendation to take HRT in the lowest dose for the shortest time, it's no wonder many physicians and the public remain confused.

WHAT ABOUT THE ALTERNATIVES?

You don't have to look far to see what a big business menopause has become. In 2022, the global menopause market was valued at nearly $17 billion, and it is expected to surpass $24 billion by 2030.[37] Everywhere, we see the explosion of websites, podcasts, telemedicine services, conferences, and new niches for the wellness industry, and the marketplace is flooded with old products packaged as new "specialized" treatments. Spas and resorts offer expensive menopause retreats that provide massages, meditation, advice, and conversation with fellow sufferers. The mainstream media, asleep at the wheel when the WHI was broadcasting its exaggerated alarms, are finally featuring stories on menopause and treatments for symptoms. We call these new treatments the ABE approach — Anything But Oestrogen — because they take advantage of women's fear of oestrogen to promote non-HRT interventions, most of which are not helpful and some of which are harmful.

A particularly cynical example is a drug that the FDA approved in 2023 to "bring relief to women struggling with the exasperating hot flashes of menopause." Fezolinetant (Veozah) is "the first drug specifically designed to reduce the frequency and severity of flushing and sweating spells that occur as a woman's oestrogen levels fall." The first drug? Hardly, but hey, it's nonhormonal. It also costs about $550 a month and has none of oestrogen's benefits for heart, bone, and other menopausal symptoms. And take a look at its side effects: abdominal pain, diarrhea, difficulty sleeping (insomnia), back pain, and...wait for it...hot flushes! A pill to cure insomnia that can cause insomnia? A pill to reduce hot flushes that causes hot flushes?

All drugs, from aspirin to Zyrtec, have side effects and potential risks, and HRT is no exception. Hormone replacement side effects may include dry eyes, vaginal discharge, and breast tenderness, symptoms that can continue in some women for as long as one year. HRT also has small but more serious risks, including gallbladder disease and blood clots in veins. (We will evaluate the balance of risks versus benefits in chapter 8.) Understandably, many women don't like taking any prescription drug unless it is medically necessary; others believe that HRT is riskier than other medication options. Let's consider them.

Some women may decide to do nothing and endure the symptoms. Others want to do something but don't want to take oestrogen, with or without progesterone, in which case they can take prescription drugs for specific menopausal symptoms or try any of the zillions of botanicals and other "natural" products marketed for menopause. We won't even discuss the ever-popular all-purpose pabulum about "individualized lifestyle modifications and non-pharmacologic therapies" such as these recommendations from the *Journal of Clinical Endocrinology and Metabolism:* Women should stop smoking, lose weight, drink less alcohol, take vitamin D and calcium, eat a healthy diet, use vaginal lubricants, and get regular physical activity. And for severe hot flushes and sleepless nights, the authors of the article added that cognitive behavioral therapy, hypnosis, and acupuncture "may be helpful."[38] All perfectly sensible advice (apart from taking vitamin D and calcium, which are mostly useless and have no benefit even for preventing fractures in postmenopausal women not taking oestrogen, as we will see in chapter 5). Unfortunately none of these approaches is more effective in alleviating menopausal symptoms than a placebo.

Some women are given gabapentin (Neurontin), a drug primarily used to treat seizures and nerve pain but increasingly used off-label for treating hot flushes. Gabapentin does help reduce them somewhat—though not as much as oestrogen does—but it doesn't help other menopause symptoms, and its side effects include (to list just a few) dizziness, drowsiness, fatigue, unsteadiness, nausea, diarrhea, constipation, headache, breast swelling, and dry mouth. Because it is a central nervous system depressant, it can amplify the effects of other central nervous system depressants, such as Ambien and Valium. In addition, it is potentially addictive and may cause withdrawal symptoms and seizures if stopped abruptly. The FDA has declined to approve either gabapentin or paroxetine for hot flushes, noting that in studies, both drugs had only marginal benefits,[39] but this detail has not deterred physicians from prescribing them off-label for women who don't want or cannot take oestrogen. Since these medications are not FDA-approved for this purpose, information about them comes only from doctors' experiences and clinical observations, which is why dosages vary, as do estimates of how long it takes for the drug to reduce hot flushes—anywhere from four weeks to three months!

Antidepressants are widely prescribed and can be effective in reducing hot flushes and insomnia. But a large review of the effectiveness of antidepressants concluded that "data on the benefits [of these medications] are conflicting."[40] And of course, antidepressants come with their own often unpleasant side effects and risks and do not relieve any other menopausal symptoms.

Women who don't want to take HRT often turn to the most widely used alternatives, namely botanicals and natural products like Chinese herbs, black cohosh, ginseng, St. John's Wort, and ginkgo biloba. Some practitioners, even those who believe that HRT is safe, suggest that women who don't want to take hormones can try a cocktail of herbs, one for this symptom and another for that one. Physicians at the Well Woman Centre in Dublin, who regard HRT as the "most effective prescription medicine for menopause," suggest that women who don't want to take hormones might consider "omega 3s for brain function, vitamin D for bones, Starflower Oil for breast tenderness. Vitamin E oil can be used for vaginal dryness."[41] Countless popular books of menopause advice recommend these herbal products, a multibillion-dollar industry, but one randomized controlled study after another finds that none of them reduces menopausal symptoms any more than placebos do. A sampling:

- The Isoflavone Clover Extract Study found that two dietary supplements derived from red clover extract (sold as Promensil and Rimostil) did not differ from placebo in reducing hot flushes or improving menopausal quality of life.[42]
- A professor of medicine at the Women's Health Clinical Research Center at the University of California, San Francisco, concluded that "there is no convincing evidence that

acupuncture, yoga, Chinese herbs, dong quai, evening primrose oil, ginseng, kava, or red clover extract improve hot
flushes."[43]

- A meta-analysis of nonhormonal therapies for hot flushes
  found that most studies have been of poor quality, making
  generalizability of limited use. These products "are not optimal choices for most women."[44]
- A trial of black cohosh, multibotanicals, and soy found no
  meaningful reduction in the number or intensity of symptoms in the women taking herbal supplements or placebo.
  Hormone therapy, however, significantly reduced symptoms.[45]
- A trial of black cohosh failed to reduce hot flushes more than
  placebo.[46]

We could keep going, but you get the picture: Over and over,
studies find that about 20 percent of women who take herbs — red
clover, soy, flaxseed, dong quai, evening primrose oil, ginseng, wild
yam, chaste tree, hops, and sage — report improvement of symptoms, which is precisely the percentage reported by women given
the placebo. (We were glad to learn that someone is studying chaste
tree, which has a long history as a counter-aphrodisiac.) One
review, after concluding that claims about the efficacy and safety of
herbs for menopause symptoms were largely unproven, warned of a
possible association between black cohosh and liver toxicity.[47] That
is why the American College of Obstetrics and Gynecology's practice guidelines explicitly note that complementary botanicals and
natural products, including over-the-counter isoflavones, Chinese
herbs, black cohosh, ginseng, St. John's wort, and ginkgo biloba,
have not been shown to be effective. Save your money.

Finally, let us consider bioidenticals. "The Truth about Hormone Therapy," an op-ed in the *Wall Street Journal* written by three physicians—Erika Schwartz, Kent Holtorf, and David Brownstein—began with an uncritical acceptance of the WHI's findings. "Hormone-replacement therapy has become a textbook example of how special interests, a confused medical establishment, and opportunists can combine to complicate the issue and deny patients access to safe and effective treatments," they wrote.[48] Fortunately, the Women's Health Initiative brought HRT to "an abrupt halt" because it "proved unequivocally that the drugs were *unsafe* and significant factors in increasing the risk of heart attacks, strokes and breast cancer in the more than 16,000 women studied." What was a woman to do? Women felt horrible when they went off HRT, and their physicians, hostages to the medical establishment, had nothing to offer except antidepressants. No worries! Bioidentical drugs to the rescue! They are identical, so they work, but not exactly identical, so they aren't harmful. Drs. Schwartz, Holtorf, and Brownstein are founding members of the Bioidentical Hormone Initiative.

How can a drug be identical but not the same? *Bioidentical* is a marketing term, and quite a brilliant one at that, because it implies that it provides all the benefits of oestrogen without...what? Oestrogen's risks? Bioidenticals, which require a prescription just as HRT does, usually contain estradiol, the predominant form of circulating oestrogen in women. (Yams contain estradiol, but don't even think about it. You'd have to eat a *lot* of yams.) Premarin contains at least ten forms of oestrogen, including estradiol, but it also has equilin, the form believed to be most beneficial in preserving brain function.[49] Nonetheless, commercially manufactured oestrogen and bioidentical oestrogen (usually estradiol) are approved and regulated by the FDA.

In contrast, *compounded* bioidentical hormones, which are widely used in the United States, are generally prepared by a local pharmacy according to a prescription written by a woman's physician. They are not standardized pharmaceutical products, they are not regulated by the FDA, and all major medical societies have discouraged their use as an alternative to approved forms of oestrogen and progesterone.[50] In 2020, the National Academies of Science confirmed the unreliability of compounded bioidentical hormones (cBHT). After 21 months of data collection and analysis, the investigating committee concluded: "Given the paucity of data on the safety and effectiveness of cBHT...there is insufficient evidence to support the overall clinical utility of cBHT as treatment for menopause."[51]

In her excellent review of the dangers of compounded bioidenticals, investigative journalist Cathryn Jakobson Ramin also cautioned against the use of implanted pellets, which became popular in the United States after the WHI scared women off HRT. Women can pay up to $3,000 a year or more at the "hormone clinics" that implant them. "No FDA-approved pharmaceutical company manufactures hormone pellets," she wrote. "In fact, only a few compounders have the equipment to make a product that won't fall apart and will dissolve slowly rather than all at once. There have been reports of poorly manufactured pellets that released staggeringly high levels of hormones to women." Wulf H. Utian, founder of the North American Menopause Society, told her, "Not only can they deliver unsafe blood levels of hormones, but they may also be impure products, carrying the danger of infection. Infection may also occur when the pellet is inserted surgically under the skin. Other than the financial reward to the compounding pharmacy and the physician, I can think of no reason to use these non-FDA-approved products."[52]

Why, then, are compounded bioidenticals still so popular? An informal focus group of 21 women who were using or had used them were asked about their reasons for avoiding conventional HRT. They mentioned fear of its risks, an aversion to "mares' urine," and, most of all, an "overarching distrust of a medical system perceived as dismissive of their concerns and overly reliant on pharmaceuticals." They also enjoyed what they regarded as the "enhanced clinical care and attention" they got from their alternative-care doctors. "We find," the researchers concluded, "that women are not only seeking alternatives to conventional pharmaceuticals, but alternatives to conventional care where their menopausal experience is solicited, their treatment goals are heard, and they are engaged as agents in managing their own menopause."[53] It seems an unfortunate trade-off: to get the kind of physician who will listen, explain, and collaborate with them, they choose risky or ineffective treatments.*

As with all over-the-counter herbs and potions, consumers need

---

* The price of choosing an alternative medicine because it sounds or feels good can be high. In 2018, the *Journal of the National Cancer Institute* reported a study of death rates from nonmetastatic cancer over a five-and-a-half-year window. The researchers compared outcomes for 280 patients who chose alternative medicine instead of chemotherapy, radiotherapy, and surgery, with 560 patients treated traditionally. The patients who relied on unproven alternatives were, on average, 2.5 times more likely to die within that time, and for some cancers, the risk associated with alternative medicine was much worse: almost six times higher for patients with breast cancer and four times higher for colon cancer. (Johnson SB, Park HS, Gross CP, Yu JB. Use of alternative medicine for cancer and its impact on survival. JNCI. 2018;110:121–24.)

to be aware of sciencey-sounding interventions that have no scientific basis, even when the advice comes from physicians who claim to be specialists in treating menopause. One such physician wrote to Avrum and commended him for his critique of the Women's Health Initiative but added that she nonetheless still opposed HRT. She herself, she said, preferred "bioidentical hormone replacement therapy (BHRT) and the Wiley Protocol," claiming they had better safety and efficacy than conventional HRT. When Av asked her for studies demonstrating that overall "safety and efficacy," she did not respond.

The Wiley Protocol is a bioidentical hormone system devised by Teresa S. Wiley, a woman with no scientific or medical credentials. Wiley claims that her method not only alleviates menopausal symptoms but also increases overall health and, who knows, may make you rich while you sleep.[54] We can't improve on Wikipedia's summary: "The protocol has been criticized by members of the medical community for the dosages of the hormones used, side effects of the treatment, potential physiologic effects, Wiley's lack of medical or clinical qualifications to design the protocol, lack of empirical evidence demonstrating it as safe or effective, ethical problems with the clinical trial that is being run to test it and potential financial conflicts of interest regarding financial incentives." Is that all?

The Take-Home

The question of whether to take HRT is no longer an issue for individual women to solve for themselves because of the economic damage to society of the numbers of midlife women reducing their work hours or leaving the workforce due to incapacitating symptoms (which, remember, can include depression, palpitations, infections, and pain as well as hot flushes). In 2020, the British Medical Association (BMA) conducted a study of 2,000 women doctors in England, finding that those "going through the menopause are reducing their hours, moving to lower-paid roles or retiring early from medicine due to sexism and ageism in surgeries and hospitals."[55]

The BMA discovered a strong pattern of highly experienced women leaving their positions as clinical leaders or directors or retiring from medicine altogether, because they were struggling to cope with severe menopause symptoms without support from management or colleagues. More than 90 percent said that their symptoms had affected their working lives, but two-fifths (38 percent) said they were unable to make the changes to their work schedules and demands that would allow them to manage their discomforts while continuing their practice. Almost half said they wanted to discuss their symptoms with their managers, yet only 16 percent had done so; the rest feared they would be "laughed at or ridiculed" if they did. For some, the stress of symptoms plus dealing with sexist employers and a rigidly structured hospital system became too much. One doctor said, "I left a job I loved." Here is another doctor's story:

> Dr Anne Carson, chair of BMA Northern Ireland's consultant committee and consultant radiologist at Craigavon area hospital, has been having menopausal symptoms for the last five years. "I never expected to have crippling menopausal symptoms—I've never not been able to deal with the

demands of my life—but the menopause hit me like a roll-ercoaster. Talking about the menopause as a doctor is taboo. I held off for two years but I was suffering chronic sleep deprivation throughout that time because my night sweats were so bad. I could only sleep for a few hours at a time before having to get up to have a shower. I was getting to the point where my decision-making ability wasn't safe, so I had no choice: I had to tell my line manager. It wasn't something I wanted to do because the stigma is so great but my line manager was actually very understanding."

Unfortunately for Dr. Carson, the National Health Service did not allow her to determine her hours and schedule. If she wanted to regulate her sleep better, her only option was to cut down her on-call hours, and that meant cutting her take-home pay, which, as a single mother, she could not afford to do.

Because menopausal women in the United Kingdom and the United States are the fastest-growing demographic in the work-place, when they reduce their hours or leave their jobs, their employers and the economy suffer. No wonder corporations are paying attention, with growing efforts at creating (and, of course, marketing and profiting from) "menopause-friendly" policies. In 2023, New York City mayor Eric Adams promised "to change the stigma around menopause in this city" and "create more menopause-friendly workplaces for our city workers through improving policies and our buildings." (Good. But if corporations truly cared about their female workers' productivity and well-being, why couldn't they manage to create child-friendly policies as well?)

We obviously welcome ways of reducing the stigma of

menopause, educating women about the most effective treatments, and making workplaces more flexible. But we also agree with Stephanie Faubion, medical director of the North American Menopause Society, who told the *New York Times*, "The last thing we need is some other reason for workplace discrimination against women and to handicap them in some way by saying there's something wrong with them at menopause that requires accommodation."[56] Faubion and Chrisandra Shufelt argued that the "menopause management vacuum" should be filled not by placebos, lounge chairs, and retreats but by educating providers (in medical school, in continuing education programs, and with professional guidelines) about menopause, female anatomy, and effective hormonal treatments; removing barriers to insurance coverage of hormonal therapies, which were based on outdated WHI claims of harm; and making the discussion of menopausal symptoms as acceptable and unstigmatized as the topic of erectile dysfunction is for men.[57]

Thus, while we agree with the feminist critique that women's life problems are often overmedicalized, we also believe that the solution is not to undermedicalize them and ignore or incorrectly treat symptoms that have clear physiological origins. The goal, surely, is what is best for an individual woman. For Katie Taylor, the solution was neither antidepressants nor quitting her demanding job; it was taking hormones. Often, after Avrum's patients begin HRT, they call him, very upset. "I had felt old and used up," one woman said, "but after being on oestrogen, the self I thought was long gone was back. I'm angry at all the time I wasted feeling miserable."

If HRT were of benefit only for women like this patient, that would be reason enough to endorse it. Indeed, as we have seen, the pendulum has begun to swing back to an acceptance of the evidence that HRT is beneficial, with very low risks, for the most severe symptoms of menopause.

Now the debate has moved to the next level: If a woman has no worrisome symptoms in menopause or did have them but they have subsided, should she take HRT to prevent future diseases and difficulties? For JoAnn Manson of the WHI, the answer is still no. The decline in the use of HRT that followed the WHI's original reports "was not optimal," she now says, because women were suffering from symptoms that disrupted sleep and impaired their quality of life, which in turn affected health. However, she added, "this does not mean that we're going back to 25 years ago where hormone therapy was used for prevention of cardiovascular disease."[58]

In chapters 4, 5, and 6 we will argue with that recommendation, because it now appears that HRT does far more than improve the quality of women's lives during menopause. It also saves lives and prolongs lives by significantly reducing the risks of heart disease, osteoporosis, colon cancer, and diabetes. But before we get there, we know we have to address the T. rex in the room: women's greatest fear, and the WHI's sole remaining assertion, that HRT increases the risk of breast cancer.

2

Does Oestrogen Cause
Breast Cancer?

A s Av began to question the received wisdom on oestrogen, he found himself in the same position as the physicians who dared question the once universal belief that the best treatment for breast cancer was radical mastectomy, an idea promoted by the surgeon William Halsted in the late nineteenth and early twentieth centuries. Radical mastectomy was based in part on Halsted's theory that breast cancer spread almost exclusively from the original site into contiguous areas. Find a tumor in the breast? Then it is essential to remove the tumor, the entire breast, and everything adjacent — a "radical" procedure.

Halsted's assumption was logical, widely accepted, and wrong. Between 1927 and 1981, 24 studies reported on more than 4,000 patients with breast cancer who had been treated with lumpectomy (removal of the tumor only) and, usually, subsequent radiation. In all but two of those studies, survival rates, even up to thirty years later, were similar to those of patients treated with variations of the radical mastectomy.[1] Randomized trials and observational studies continue to show that breast-conserving surgery is almost always as effective in terms of disease-free survival and often better. Yet rates of mastectomies, especially bilateral mastectomies, for treatment of localized breast cancer have been rising since 2006—another manifestation of the fear associated with breast cancer. In the overwhelming majority of these cases, mastectomy is not indicated and not recommended. Yet many patients panic and say, "Just take it off—take them both off so I don't have to worry." They would rather cope with the pain, discomfort, prolonged recovery, and physical impairments of extensive surgery than deal with anxiety, even though the more extensive surgery does not offer a greater chance for cure.

Like Halsted's mistaken notion that breast cancer spreads *only* through adjacent areas (rather than through the bloodstream), the belief that oestrogen causes breast cancer is logical, widely accepted, and wrong. Consider these findings:

If oestrogen were an important cause of breast cancer, we would expect rates of breast cancer to decline after menopause, when oestrogen levels naturally diminish. Instead, breast cancer rates increase, even in women not taking HRT.

If oestrogen were carcinogenic, we would hardly expect it to be beneficial for women with breast cancer. After all, you would not treat patients with lung cancer by dramatically increasing the number of cigarettes they smoke daily. But high doses of oestrogen have been used to treat metastatic breast cancer, and women diagnosed with breast cancer while on HRT or oestrogen alone often have a better prognosis than those who are not taking it.

If oestrogen were carcinogenic, a woman's lifetime cumulative level of oestrogen would be a major contributor to breast cancer. But that idea, still held by many physicians, is based on weak and largely circumstantial evidence. It came from the perception that women who enter menarche very early and who have late menopause have a higher risk of breast cancer, because they have allegedly been exposed to more years of oestrogen. But they don't. Four separate studies have examined the breast cancer risk in women who started their periods between the ages of 12 and 17 and women whose periods started at age 11 or younger. Two of these studies reported no differences in risk. The other two found a significant reduction in risk only among women who started their periods at age 17 and older, a very small percentage of the population.[2] Moreover, because the endometrium (the lining of the uterus) is more sensitive to oestrogen than the breast, then the risk of endometrial cancer should also be related to early menarche and late menopause. It is not.

If oestrogen were carcinogenic, pregnancy, during which circulating oestrogen concentrations are at least ten times higher than they are at other periods of a woman's life, should raise the risk of breast cancer. But it doesn't. In 1991, Mitchell Gail and Jacques Benichou of the National Cancer Institute observed that because pregnancy markedly elevates levels of oestrogen and progesterone, women who have their first child when they are young and go on to have many children should be at the highest risk of developing breast cancer. Actually, they have the lowest risk.[3] A full-term pregnancy before age 20 reduces lifetime breast cancer risk by 70 percent.[4] Women who are diagnosed with breast cancer during pregnancy have a prognosis similar to nonpregnant women at the same stage of breast cancer. According to an international collaborative study, pregnancy *following* treatment of breast cancer had no negative effect on prognosis after a median follow-up of 7.2 years, even for women with oestrogen-receptor-positive [ER+] tumors.[5] Another international study of 1,252 breast cancer patients with BRCA mutations reported no increased risk of breast cancer recurrence associated with pregnancy.[6] Further, terminating the pregnancies in women with recently diagnosed breast cancer, thereby eliminating the increased level of circulating oestrogen, produced no benefit for either the disease's course or its prognosis.[7]

One of the most surprising and important studies of pregnancy and breast cancer appeared in 2023. Medical oncologist Ann Partridge and her colleagues conducted an international study of 497 women treated for ER+ breast cancer.[8] The women were, per the usual procedure for treating breast cancer, receiving therapy designed to suppress oestrogen's effects. But Partridge allowed them to suspend that treatment for two years if they wished to become pregnant. Nearly half of these women had in vitro fertilization, which greatly elevates oestrogen and progesterone levels, and in the ensuing three years, 507 became pregnant. Partridge compared them with women who had continued their oestrogen-suppressing treatment. After three years, there was no difference in the risk of breast cancer recurrence.

Many women diagnosed with ER+ breast cancer assume, understandably, that oestrogen is feeding the kind of breast cancer they have. But it isn't. Normal breast cells have receptors for oestrogen on their cell membranes. If that receptor is discovered on the membrane of a breast cancer cell, it usually means the breast cancer is growing slowly enough to adopt this normal cell characteristic.

·Indeed, in most breast cancers, ER+ cells are *not* the ones proliferating. A similar receptor has been identified for progesterone. The
presence of oestrogen receptors or progesterone receptors on the
surface of a breast cancer cell does not mean that the breast cancer
was *caused* by oestrogen or progesterone. In fact, the cells of early
breast cancer and the ones that multiply within breast cancer are
generally oestrogen-receptor- and progesterone-receptor-negative.[9]

*　　*　　*

So, does oestrogen cause breast cancer? Conjectures and controversies have swirled around this question for more than a hundred years,
and that provides a clue to the answer. The Nobel Prize–winning
physicist Richard Feynman had a good test for truth in science: "If
something is true, really so," he said, "if you continue observations
and improve the effectiveness of the observations, the effects stand
out more obviously."[10] If you continue your observations and all you
get are muddy and inconsistent answers, something is wrong with
your method or, more likely, with your hypothesis.

Advances in science are rarely achieved by one dramatic insight
or experimental finding. They are usually the result of small steps
and conclusions, many of which point in the same general direction,
allowing the evolution of an idea that can then be tested and either
verified or disproved. Unfortunately, not all scientists are as dispas-
sionate in their pursuit of a finding as Feynman was. For him,
being wrong was as informative as being right. But many scientists,
like almost all mortals, would rather be right; and some are willing
to bend their experiments' findings to fit their theories.

Efforts to understand and treat breast cancer have a long history.[11] In the late 1800s, a few physicians suggested there might be

a causal relationship between a product of the ovary, most likely oestrogen, and the development and progression of breast cancer. In 1882, Thomas William Nunn reported the case history of a perimenopausal woman with breast cancer whose disease regressed six months after her periods stopped. In 1889, Albert Schinzinger, observing that breast cancer was less aggressive in older women than in younger women, proposed that removing both ovaries in premenopausal women with breast cancer would send them into early menopause and thus cause the breast cancer to regress. Schinzinger never performed the surgery, however, because he was unable to convince his colleagues (or his patients) of its potential merit. But six years later, in 1895, George Thomas Beatson removed both ovaries of a woman who had extensive, recurrent breast cancer. The patient's tumor regressed completely and she survived for four years after the surgery. One year later, Stanley Boyd, an English surgeon, removed both ovaries in a woman with metastatic breast cancer; she survived for twelve years after her surgery. Boyd later wrote, "My working hypothesis is that internal secretion of the ovaries in some cases favors the growth of the cancer."

There matters stood for almost half a century.

After the development of Premarin in 1942, the rising popularity of oestrogen in the 1950s and 1960s was tempered by the discovery in the 1970s that the incidence of endometrial cancer, a generally curable cancer of the cells lining the uterus, was increased four to eight times in women taking oestrogen alone.[12] Fortunately, the addition of progesterone, another female hormone, not only negated the increased risk of uterine cancer but actually protected against it; women taking progesterone with oestrogen had a lower incidence of endometrial cancer than women who received no hormones.[13] That is why, since the early 1980s, most women who start hormone therapy after a hysterectomy get oestrogen alone, while women who still have a uterus receive oestrogen plus progesterone.

Today, the major concern about the possible risks of hormones is not uterine cancer but breast cancer. As Avrum pored over the research conducted throughout the 1980s and 1990s, a drumbeat of reassuring studies greeted him. Here's a sample:

- 1986: No statistically significant increased risk of breast cancer among women on Premarin, even among those who had been taking it for more than twenty years.[14]
- 1988: No association between oestrogen alone and breast cancer.[15]
- 1991: No association between oestrogen alone and breast cancer.[16]
- 1991: No increased risk of breast cancer among Premarin users even after fifteen years of use.[17]
- 1992: In a study of women randomly assigned to take placebo or HRT and followed for twenty-two years, researchers found that 11.5 percent of women taking the placebo developed breast cancer—but *none* of the women on HRT did.[18]
- 1995: Compared to women who had never taken HRT, women who took HRT for eight or more years had a reduced risk of breast cancer.[19]
- 1995: In the Nurses' Health Study, which followed 121,700 female registered nurses from 1976 through 1992, women who had ever been on HRT, even for more than ten years, had no increased risk of breast cancer compared to women who had never taken HRT.[20]

- 1997: Among 41,837 Iowa women between ages 55 and 69, those taking HRT did not have an increased risk of breast cancer. This was also true for women who had a family history of breast cancer.[21]

But more stunning and counterintuitive discoveries about oestrogen and breast cancer were to come from studies of women with deleterious BRCA1 and BRCA2 mutations, which are associated with an increased risk of ovarian and of breast cancer. BRCA-positive women are usually advised to have both ovaries removed, because that dramatically reduces the risk of ovarian cancer and cuts the risk of breast cancer in half. If lowered oestrogen levels following removal of the ovaries were the reason for the drop in breast cancer risk, then giving these women oestrogen to alleviate symptoms of menopause would be illogical; indeed, it would be dangerous. Incredibly, it isn't.

Epidemiologist Timothy Rebbeck and his colleagues studied 462 pre- and postmenopausal women with the BRCA1 and BRCA2 mutations. They compared BRCA-positive women who had been taking oestrogen only or HRT for a few years following removal of their ovaries with those who had never taken hormones. They found no increased risk of breast cancer.[22] Neither did medical oncologist Andrea Eisen, who studied 472 BRCA1-positive postmenopausal women, half of whom were taking hormones and half of whom were not. "Among postmenopausal women with a BRCA1 mutation," she wrote, "oestrogen use, which averaged around four years, was not associated with an increased risk of breast cancer; *indeed, in this population, it was associated with a significant decreased risk.*"[23] (Our italics.) A later study replicated this counterintuitive conclusion. Again, women with a BRCA1 mutation who had been on HRT for an average of 4.3 years had no increased risk of breast cancer.[24]

As early as 1987, a consensus-development conference concluded that "well-defined epidemiological studies [of oestrogen therapy] do not suggest an overall increase in the risk of breast cancer in postmenopausal women."[25] And a 1993 editorial in the *New England Journal of Medicine* (*NEJM*) recommended that "all postmenopausal women be considered candidates for hormone replacement therapy and be educated about its risks and benefits."[26]

*   *   *

At this point, you are either saying to yourself, "Why would anyone ever think that oestrogen increases the risk of breast cancer?" or "But wait! What aren't you telling me about the risks of hormones?" Good questions both.

Those who make the case against hormones cite two studies in particular. One was published in 1989 in the *NEJM* by a team of eminent researchers led by Leif Bergkvist and Hans-Olov Adami at University Hospital, Uppsala, Sweden. It reported a 440 percent increased risk of breast cancer among women who had been on HRT.[27] Pretty frightening, right?

Let's look closer at that study. The researchers analyzed prescription forms for oestrogen alone or HRT for the entire female population around Uppsala, more than 23,000 women. But rather than going through every single record, which would have been a time-consuming challenge, they selected a subgroup, one in every 30 or so women, ending up with 638 women who filled out two sequential questionnaires. There was no increased risk of breast cancer among women taking oestrogen alone. Among an unspecified, smaller number of the 638 women who were taking HRT, the authors calculated that 2.2 breast cancers would be expected; instead, there were 10 cases. And that was the 440 percent increase in risk. With numbers that small, the increase could have been a statistical fluke, and in fact the researchers admitted that their result was not statistically significant—meaning it was not worth writing home about. But because this was the lead article in the *NEJM*, many physicians trumpeted that "increased risk" as if it were momentous. In a study published not long after their first one, the same authors reported that breast cancer patients who were on oestrogen at the time of diagnosis had a better prognosis than those who were not.[28] This got no media attention at all.

In an editorial accompanying that first paper, Elizabeth Barrett-Connor, a biomedical scientist, wrote: "For the average North American woman, who will be postmenopausal for one third of her life, the benefits of oestrogen seem strongly established. In my opinion, the data are not conclusive enough to warrant any immediate change in the way we approach hormone replacement."[29] The *Harvard Medical School Health Letter* also reviewed the Swedish study and concluded that the difference between 2.2 and 10 cases of breast cancer was too small to provide a statistically stable result, let alone one that warranted overturning most of the earlier research that "has given us no reason to expect a strong association between oestrogen replacement and breast cancer."[30]

The second big study cited by those opposing HRT was published in 1997 in the prestigious British journal the *Lancet*. This was the Collaborative Reanalysis, a survey of 51 epidemiological studies from twenty-one countries involving 52,705 women with breast cancer and 108,411 women without breast cancer. Because of the study's enormous size and the sterling reputation of its more than twenty collaborators, it is still frequently cited as one of *the* definitive investigations of hormones and breast cancer. The researchers — led by epidemiologists Richard Doll, Richard Peto, and Valerie Beral of the project's analysis and writing committee — reported no increase in breast cancer among women who had taken HRT in the past, no matter how long they had taken it.[31] Did the researchers then say, "Good news!" and move on? No; they reanalyzed their voluminous data to see if they could find, anywhere, a subgroup of women who showed an increased risk of breast cancer associated with HRT. They got it by extracting the women who were still on HRT at the time they were interviewed and who had been on it for five or more years. How much of an increase did they find? Even in this artificially constructed subsample, the increased number of breast cancers in 100 women taking oestrogen for ten or more years was 0.6, less than one additional case.[32]

And that's where matters stood until 2002.

Enter the Women's Health Initiative

The WHI's announcement that HRT increases the risk of breast cancer set off fireworks and fears. The WHI followed what is considered the gold standard of scientific research, the double-blind study, in which participants are randomly assigned to take the treatment being studied or a placebo, and no one, neither the participants nor the investigators, knows who is getting which. This method is ideal for studying oestrogen because if you simply compared women who chose to take oestrogen with those who chose not to—as many earlier studies did—and found that oestrogen was beneficial, you would not be able to say whether oestrogen made women healthier or if healthier women took oestrogen.

The WHI investigators reported that women who were randomly assigned to take oestrogen on its own had had no increased risk of breast cancer. Those who still had a uterus and were assigned to take the combination of oestrogen and progestin (HRT) had a small increased risk of breast cancer (of 1.26) when compared with women who were randomly assigned to a placebo.[33] That number, 1.26, means a 26 percent increase in risk. Few noticed this sentence: "The 26 percent increase in breast cancer incidence among the HRT group compared with the placebo group almost reached nominal statistical significance." *Almost* means it did *not* reach statistical significance, and that means it could have been a spurious association. (Scientists have arbitrarily agreed that the results of a study are not considered statistically significant unless the probability that its results are due to chance alone is less than one in 20.) *Nominal* is a potentially confusing label meaning a simple, unadjusted analysis that does not consider factors that can create a false positive result for a given outcome. Of course, any increase might be of legitimate concern and warrant further investigation. Yet many reporters and physicians treated that 26 percent increase in risk as being not only statistically significant but also medically significant.

The WHI researchers continued to follow the women from the original study, updating their data as the participants stayed healthy or developed illnesses. A year later, in 2003, they reported that the small difference in breast cancer incidence between patients randomized to HRT and those randomized to placebo had narrowed, but it now barely achieved statistical significance. Still, they asserted that their 2002 report "confirmed that combined oestrogen plus progestin use increases the risk of invasive breast cancer."[34] Confirmed? *Invasive?* Well . . . not so fast.

In 2006, Garnet Anderson, co–principal investigator and biostatistician for the WHI Clinical Coordinating Center, claimed the study had demonstrated that "breast cancer rates were markedly increased among women assigned to the oestrogen plus progestin group."[35] Markedly? Even if this finding had been statistically significant, which it was not, it would have meant that HRT increased the risk of breast cancer from 5 women in one hundred to 6 in one hundred. In the WHI's press release, Anderson justified her statistical decisions this way: "Because breast cancer is so serious an event, we set the bar lower to monitor for it. We pre-specified that the change in cancer rates did not have to be that large to warrant stopping the trial. And the trial was stopped at the first clear indication of increased risk."

In other words: *We set the bar low enough to monitor for nonsignificant results if we could squeak out any.*

Yet in that same 2006 article, Anderson and colleagues reported no increased risk of breast cancer among those same women randomized to HRT. The alleged increased risk — the one worth stopping the study for — *had completely vanished.* This news did not make headlines. As the science writer Tara Parker-Pope wryly observed, the WHI "seemed to have a different standard for bad hormone news than it did for good hormone news."[36]

In 2010 the WHI authors published yet another article, this one claiming that women who had been on HRT suffered more deaths from breast cancer (2.6 versus 1.3 deaths per 10,000 women per year) than those who had been on a placebo — again, a difference that was not statistically significant.[37]

The WHI was heralded as being truly representative of women during and after menopause, and the WHI investigators repeatedly stated that all of the women they recruited were healthy at the outset of the study, but neither assertion was true. Fully 35 percent of the women were considerably overweight, and another 34 percent were obese; nearly 36 percent were being treated for high blood pressure; nearly half were either current or past cigarette smokers.[38] Moreover, the median age of participants was 63, considerably past menopause. Therefore, there is no credible reason for generalizing from the results of this study to the entire population of menopausal women.

Over the years, medical researchers have become more vocal in their critiques of the WHI's methods, findings, and conclusions. As one notable example, in 2014, Samuel Shapiro and his colleagues conducted an in-depth statistical analysis and concluded that "the over-interpretation and misrepresentation of the findings in the WHI study has resulted in major damage to the health and well-being of menopausal women. The WHI was not 'a victory for women and their health,' and the claim that 'the findings do not support the use of this therapy for chronic disease prevention' is not defensible. Nor can the pejorative editorial statement that 'the WHI overturned medical dogma regarding menopausal hormone therapy' be defended."[39]

But the most damning indictment of the WHI came from one of its principal investigators. In 2017, epidemiologist Robert Langer wrote: "Highly unusual circumstances prevailed when the WHI trial was stopped prematurely in July 2002. The investigators most capable of correcting the critical misinterpretations of the data were actively excluded from the writing and dissemination activities." *Actively excluded.* The paper of initial results, he said, was written by a small group in the WHI program office who submitted it to *JAMA* without informing the principal investigators. He described what happened at the meeting of the principal investigators and the NIH program staff:

> The investigator group was stunned by the announcement that the Data Safety and Monitoring Committee had recommended stopping the oestrogen-progestin trial and that the director had accepted their recommendation. Minutes later the group was shocked by the distribution of a typeset copy of the primary results paper soon to be published in *JAMA. This was the first time that the vast majority of principal investigators had seen the paper.* [Our italics.] The meeting was paused so that we could read it. Some of us were aghast. Concerns were raised about the propriety of producing a paper on behalf of the entire study group in this manner. More importantly, concerns were raised about the tone, the analyses conducted and reported, and the interpretation of the results in the paper.[40]

The protesting investigators were allowed to do some quick editing of the article before lunch, addressing its "tone and interpretation," and the changes were sent by courier to *JAMA*. They were too late. The courier returned to tell them that the issue had already been printed and was in the warehouses ready to be mailed out.

In short, the procedure violated key scientific conventions: statistical accuracy, co-author review, and publication in a professional journal *before* the hoopla of press releases and other publicity. Jacques Rossouw, a cardiologist who was leading the WHI, told Parker-Pope that the WHI "was intentionally going for 'high impact' when it called the press conference," because they didn't want their news to "get lost in the shuffle of daily news events," especially when their goal "was to shake up the medical establishment and change the thinking about hormones."[41]

And that is the giveaway. Far from setting out to do an unbiased study to investigate the possible benefits and risks of hormones for women during and after menopause, far from their disingenuous claims that they fully expected to learn that hormones were safe, some of the principal investigators had an agenda from the outset: to "change the thinking about hormones" and show that they were harmful. After the WHI had begun but six years before any findings were published, Rossouw had published a paper in which he lamented the widespread use of oestrogen.[42] "The bandwagon [in support of oestrogen replacement therapy] is clearly rolling," he wrote, "as anyone who reads newspapers or magazines, watches television, or talks to colleagues can attest. The bandwagon appears to be picking up in speed and volume. The putative benefits of HRT are being trumpeted to postmenopausal women, with only transient muting for reports of possible adverse effects." It is time, Rossouw argued, to put "the brakes on that bandwagon." The WHI certainly did.

The WHI and *JAMA* might have been justified in bypassing scientific conventions if the findings were truly of enormous medical import, but they were not. Instead, the investigators collaborated in generating international panic based on data and conclusions that were open to serious question. Why did they do this? We get this question all the time, and we don't know. In 2002, a few months after the WHI's first stop-the-presses report was published, Rowan Chlebowski, one of its investigators, spoke about the study at the continuing medical education program that Av was running at his hospital. The physicians in the audience were not impressed by the statistically nonsignificant evidence being presented, and the following exchange occurred during the question-and-answer period:

Physician: About your claim of the increased risk of breast cancer for women on HRT, I'm not an oncologist so this might be a stupid question. I was under the impression that if the confidence interval [a measure of a finding's strength] included the number one, that it was not particularly meaningful.

Chlebowski: Yeah, yeah, you know, that's right. And you know what happens? What happens is, if it's an important question and if it's a big study ... and you can't do it again because it costs too much money, then they'll say that's the best data there is and then [inaudible] the statistical police have to leave the room. So that's the answer.

Translation: We won't ever be able to do this study again. We know, we just know in our heart of hearts, that HRT is harmful and causes breast cancer. And even if it doesn't cause cancer so much, it causes other diseases for sure. Therefore, if we get ambiguous answers or nonsignificant ones, we ask the statistical police to leave the room.

Chlebowski has not modified his position since. On the contrary, every few years he publishes another paper repeating the same argument defending the WHI's claims of HRT's risks and harms. The latest as we write this, published in 2023 with Aaron K. Aragaki, claims that HRT increases women's risk of developing breast cancer, though not of dying of breast cancer.[43] The WHI's 2002 warning that HRT caused breast cancer, they wrote, had saved thousands of lives. How? Because the number of women taking hormones immediately plummeted, and so did rates of breast cancer. Ergo, oestrogen causes breast cancer, and stopping oestrogen prevents women from getting breast cancer, which could kill them. They ignored their own evidence that HRT does not increase the risk of death from breast cancer.

This assertion has three fundamental flaws. First, according to CDC statistics, the decline in breast cancer incidence in the United States was evident as early as 1999, three years *before* the release of the WHI's initial results.[44] The decline was reported among white but not Black women, and there was no decline in breast cancer rates in many Western countries that also experienced dramatic declines in HRT prescriptions, among them Austria, Belgium, Denmark, England, Finland, Germany, Ireland, Israel, the Netherlands, Norway, Scotland, Sweden, and Switzerland.[45] Second, breast cancer incidence rates in the United States have increased by roughly 0.5 percent annually since the premature termination of the WHI's trial in 2002, even though hormone use has remained low;[46] according to the FDA, in 2023, 82 percent of American women over 45 reported at least one menopausal symptom, but only 10.5 percent had used any form of menopausal hormone therapy.[47] And third, breast cancer usually takes from 9 to 16 years to become clinically identifiable.[48] How, then, could a drop in the rate of breast cancer be related to stopping HRT six months to one year prior? It is not biologically plausible.

Chlebowski and his colleagues tried to wriggle out of that problem by saying that because when women went off oestrogen, they removed a stimulus to the growth of *already present but not yet detectable* (subclinical) breast cancer.[49] If that were so, the decreased national incidence should have been confined to small, early, non-invasive breast cancers; it was not. It occurred almost entirely with invasive breast cancers.[50] We don't know whether to laugh or cry at the WHI's persistent inconsistencies and tangled reasoning as they remain determined to convince the world that HRT causes breast cancer. On the one hand, they take credit for having saved lives because the incidence of breast cancer decreased soon after they warned women away from HRT—as if breast cancer could develop in six months. On the other hand, they reported an increased incidence of breast cancer among the women who were long off HRT, even after seventeen years of follow-up.[51]

All of this tap-dancing is intended to disguise the major statistical mistake the WHI made: The investigators misinterpreted their own data and they knew this as early as 2006. Women randomly assigned to take HRT did not have a *higher* rate of breast cancer; the placebo group had an unusually *low* rate—possibly because many of them had been on hormones before they entered the study. When they were removed from comparison, there was no longer a difference in breast cancer rates between the HRT group and the control group.[52] Chlebowski and his colleagues have consistently ignored this crucial reinterpretation of their own findings.

In light of the accumulating reports by senior WHI investigators confirming the survival benefits of oestrogen, we were dismayed by the inaccurate statement in a *New York Times* letter to the editor by Cynthia A. Thomson and Garnet Anderson on behalf of the WHI Steering Committee. The worldwide decrease in the use of menopausal hormone therapy, in response to the WHI's claims of risk, they wrote, "undoubtedly has saved millions of lives and billions of US healthcare dollars."[53] This enthusiastic assertion is even less valid today than it was in 2014, when Anderson joined other WHI investigators in celebrating a postulated $35.2 billion net economic return from the WHI trials.[54] On the contrary, data have shown that the fear generated by the WHI has actually *increased* mortality, especially among hysterectomized women denied oestrogen treatment and among older women dying of heart disease and hip fracture;[55] it has also *increased* health-care spending.[56]

*   *   *

For readers who are gluttons for evidence and wish to learn more about which risks are "riskiest" and how they are assessed, read on.

ENTER THE MILLION WOMEN STUDY: RUMMAGING FOR RISKS

A year after the WHI exploded onto the medical landscape, another enormous project generated headlines that added to women's worries. The Million Women Study reported an increased risk of breast cancer in British women taking oestrogen or HRT.[57] It wasn't a million women and it wasn't really a study, but its dramatic heading generated widespread attention.

In Britain, women are able to get a free routine breast screening every three years, courtesy of the National Health Service. Taking advantage of this large population, the Million Women Study sent each individual with a mammogram appointment—yes, a million of them—a letter and questionnaire, asking about their hormone use and any diagnoses of breast cancer. Three years later, they followed up with a second questionnaire; fewer than half of the women responded to both. The total incidence of breast cancer was 1 percent among oestrogen-only users and 1.4 percent among HRT users. Of that tiny percentage, the increased risk appeared in current users but not past users, even if the past use had exceeded fifteen years. Moreover, the average time from joining the "study" to diagnosis of breast cancer was only 1.2 years; the median time from diagnosis to death from breast cancer was only 1.7 years. Given the lengthy lag time for breast cancer to become detectable, as we noted, it is more likely that the breast cancers were not directly related to HRT use and were already present, though undiagnosed, at the time the women first enrolled.

*   *   *

The WHI and the Million Women Study, like many other efforts to identify the causes of disease, committed two statistical errors. One involves how risks are reported; the other involves a statistical manipulation called *data mining*. Stay with us here, because this information could improve your life—and maybe even save it.

Consider the difference between absolute risk and relative risk. The media, following the example of many researchers, tend to report relative risks, which are expressed in percentages that can seem more important than they are. For example, if you learn that the relative risk of breast cancer is increased by 300 percent in women who eat a bagel every morning, that sounds serious, but it is not informative. You would need to know the baseline absolute number of new breast cancer patients in women who avoid bagels. If the number of new cases in bagel-avoiders was 1 in 10,000 women and the number of new cases in bagel-eaters was 3 in 10,000 women, that *is* a 300 percent increase, but it is very likely a random result—enjoy your bagel! If the risk jumped from 100 new cases in 10,000 bagel-avoiders to 300 new cases in 10,000 bagel-eaters, also a 300 percent increase, you might reasonably be concerned and cut down on your bagel consumption.

In epidemiological studies, which generally include tens of thousands of people, it is easy to find a small relationship that may be considered significant by statistical convention but that, in practical terms, means little or nothing because of the low absolute numbers. This is why scientists who are working to promote statistical literacy, especially by helping the public and physicians understand actual versus inflated risks of diseases and treatments, emphasize that knowing the baseline of absolute numbers when comparing two groups is essential.[58] Throughout this book, we too report results that showed such-and-such a reduction (or increase) in risk, but we have taken pains wherever possible to ensure that these numbers reflect meaningful findings in absolute terms, not trivial ones. Thus, we will not cite a study if it reported a 33 percent reduction in risk if that reduction was from 3 to 2. We say "wherever possible" because, regrettably, sometimes it isn't possible to know the absolute numbers in a study because the researchers do not include them.

Many studies of HRT and risk of disease, especially breast cancer, have produced statistically modest or borderline results that have been made to look more impressive than they really are because researchers report only relative risks. In 2003, the WHI claimed that HRT increased women's risk of breast cancer by 24 percent; in 2002, it was 26 percent. Does that percentage really merit concern? The table on the next two pages lists the reported decreases and increases in relative risks associated not only with hormone therapy but also with many other things. If the relative risk is less than 1 (as it is for stress, aspirin, and coffee), it means the risk is decreased. If the relative risk is more than 1 (as it is for chewing betel quid or taking a multivitamin), it means an increased risk. You can see at a glance how weak and probably meaningless these associations are. One study finds that grapefruit reduces risk; another that it increases risk. The WHI's claims of the risks of HRT fall way below the "risks" of having an extra weekly serving of French fries in childhood, being left-handed, or being an Icelandic flight attendant, which is apparently riskier than being a Finnish flight attendant. All of these findings were published in peer-reviewed medical journals; none warranted press conferences or warnings to the public. To put them in perspective, the last entry is a truly important and meaningful link: the one between tobacco smoking and lung cancer.

Risk Factors Reportedly Associated with Breast Cancer[59]

Risk Factor	Relative Risk*
Dietary fiber intake	0.31
Significant weight gain from age 21 to present	0.52
Garlic and onions 7 to 10 times/week	0.52
High level of stress	0.60
Grapefruit	0.60
Fish oil	0.68
Large body build at menarche	0.69
Conjugated equine oestrogen (Premarin)	0.77
Aspirin	0.80
Coffee consumption >5 cups/day	0.80
Above average weight at the age of 12	0.85
Low income	0.85
Fish intake	1.14
Birth length > 20 inches	1.17
Use of antihypertensive medication for more than 5 years	1.18
Multivitamin use	1.19
Exposure to light at night	1.22
Premarin/progestin (WHI, 2003)	1.24
Premarin/progestin (WHI, 2002)	1.26
Alcohol	1.26
French fries (1 additional serving per week during preschool years)	1.27
Physical abuse in adulthood	1.28
Grapefruit (again)	1.30
Digoxin (current users)	1.39
Night-shift work	1.51
More than 15 kg weight gain during pregnancy	1.61

Flight attendant (Finnish)	1.87
Father at least 40 years old at patient's birth (premenopausal breast cancer)	1.90
Exposed to Dutch famine, 1944–1945, only between ages 2 and 9 at the time	2.01
Placental weight	2.05
Antibiotic use more than 1,001 days	2.07
Increased carbohydrate intake	2.22
Calcium-channel blocker for more than 10 years	2.40
Left-handedness (premenopausal)	2.41
Flight attendant (Icelandic)	4.10
Betel-quid chewing	4.78
Electric-blanket use	4.90

And here's a statistical association that actually means something:

Tobacco smoking and lung cancer	**26.07**

* A relative risk of 1 means there is no effect on risk. A relative risk of less than 1 means an associated decreased risk, and a relative risk of greater than 1 means an increased risk.

Another way of misrepresenting findings comes from the practice, severely frowned upon in research, of retrospective substratification, commonly known as data mining. Data mining occurs when researchers, having failed to find a statistically significant association that they had hypothesized would exist between a possible risk factor and a disease, go back into their data and rummage around, looking for other factors that might show a statistical link. This effort might yield interesting questions or hypotheses for future research, but the problem is that in a data set of many thousands of people, some relationships that are unearthed retrospectively will turn out to be statistically significant but meaningless. In *Against the Gods: The Remarkable Story of Risk,* the economist Peter Bernstein put it this way: "If you torture the data long enough, the numbers will prove anything you want."[60]

A now-famous example of the spurious results that can emerge from data mining can be seen in an article that was submitted to the *Lancet* in 1988. It reported that men hospitalized for acute heart attacks who had been taking a daily aspirin had a better survival rate than similar men who had not been on aspirin. This was obviously an important finding, and the editors agreed to accept this article with one condition: the authors would have to retrospectively substratify the 17,187 men in their study according to a variety of factors, including the men's ages, weights, and races.

Now, it would certainly be good to know if the benefit of taking aspirin (or any other drug) is affected by being old, overweight, Italian, a yoga practitioner, an owner of a 1968 red Camaro, or other demographic factors. But the authors correctly refused to do this reanalysis, explaining that it would be bad science and that the benefit or risk for these subcategories would best be assessed by a new prospective study.[61] The editors insisted: no substratification, no publication.

Backs against the editorial wall, the authors eventually turned in a revised article with the additional findings, plus one more: a slight adverse effect of aspirin on mortality in patients born under the astrological signs of Gemini and Libra in contrast to a strikingly beneficial effect of aspirin for patients born under all other astrological signs. The editors agreed to publish the article if the astrological results were omitted. "You wanted retrospective substratification, we gave you retrospective substratification," the authors said (in effect), and they demanded that the journal stick to the deal. And so this landmark article was published, explaining aspirin's effect on "myocardial infarct mortality" among men born under the signs of Gemini and Libra, the latter subgroup analysis clearly not being taken seriously in the article.[62] One scientist titled his commentary on this study "Subgroup analyses in clinical trials: Fun to look at—but don't believe them!" He wrote: "Of course most physicians (but not all!) laughed when they were presented with these results. However, when presented with other less ridiculous subgroup analyses they are likely to believe the results, and forget the example from astrology, particularly if the result can be justified by some pet theory."[63]

Here's how researchers who have the best of intentions—and a pet theory—can get caught up in data mining. Even the highly respected Nurses' Health Study, referred to earlier, made this mistake. The Nurses' Health Study, which followed more than 121,000 nurses for nearly two decades, reported no increase in breast cancer among the women who had used HRT at any point, even if they'd been on it for more than ten years. Instead of being satisfied, the investigators substratified their patients into two groups: (1) women who had been taking hormones for at least five years and were still doing so, and (2) women who had taken hormones in the past and had stopped. This time they found an increased risk of breast cancer, but only among women who were currently taking hormones and had been doing so for at least five years.[64] The Million Women Study likewise reported, through data mining, an increased risk only for current users but not past users.

If you are thinking, *Huh?* right about now, you are not alone. If oestrogen is a major risk factor in breast cancer, why would having taken it for years not be a problem but taking it at the time of the study be a risk? Think for a moment how unlikely this is. If, as many of those who oppose the use of HRT believe, *lifetime* exposure to oestrogen is associated with an increasing risk of breast cancer—the more oestrogen, the higher the risk—how can you get an increased risk among a group of women who have taken hormones for five years but not among those who took it for more than ten years? Can you think of any other documented cause of cancer (for example, tobacco or asbestos) that carries more risk if you are currently exposed to it and have been for a relatively brief time and less risk if you are not currently exposed to it but you were for many years in the past? Neither can we. That is what data mining gives you.

Consider this study from the National Cancer Institute, a follow-up of 2,082 women with breast cancer, which also had found no increase in risk associated with oestrogen alone. The increased risk associated with HRT was restricted to those who used hormones during the four years prior to diagnosis *and* who weighed 90 pounds or less. That's what data mining gives you.[65]

Or how about the finding in the table that using an electric blanket increases the risk of breast cancer? That finding was significant only for Black women, only if they used electric blankets for more than ten years—and only when those who used blankets for more than six months per year were excluded! That's what data mining gives you.

Some investigators who believe that the relative risks of HRT are serious enough to warrant concern acknowledge that the absolute risks from this treatment are small, increasing a woman's risk by no more than 2 percent.[66] Even if HRT increases the risk of breast cancer by this modest fraction, other research suggests that women on HRT live longer than those not taking it and have a lower death rate from breast cancer.[67] How can the very hormones that allegedly increase the risk of breast cancer also be responsible for better survival from that cancer?

Does Oestrogen Cause Breast Cancer? How Would We Know?

In medicine, as in law, causation is often difficult to prove beyond a reasonable doubt. A bullet fired through the brain or the heart of an otherwise healthy human being who dies shortly thereafter generally provides both a necessary and sufficient explanation for the cause of death. But many causes of disease and death are not as straightforward; they are inferred and then must be tested and confirmed — or rejected.

Consider the effort to find the cause of tuberculosis. Because tuberculosis was often concentrated in large metropolitan areas, physicians originally believed it was caused by the stress of living in crowded, noisy spaces. Accordingly, throughout the United States and Europe, tuberculosis sanitariums were set up to remove affected individuals from their allegedly stressful environments. In these peaceful retreats, patients were even placed in dark rooms with window shades lowered to further decrease stress. Thomas Mann's *The Magic Mountain* describes just such an environment.

In 1872 Robert Koch demonstrated unequivocally that the cause of tuberculosis was the tubercle bacillus, and only then were the sanitariums gradually closed and antibiotics developed to treat this scourge. To prove the role of the tubercle bacillus, Koch set up four postulates, and these have served as a template for the study of the causes of other human diseases.[68] Koch's postulates — the steps needed to demonstrate that microorganism A is indeed the cause of disease B — were as follows:

- The microorganism must be found in all organisms suffering from the disease.
- The microorganism must be isolated from a diseased organism and grown in pure culture.
- The cultured microorganism should cause the disease when introduced into a healthy organism.
- The microorganism must be re-isolated from the inoculated diseased host and shown to be the same as the original causative agent.

This causal *chain of evidence* is now an established format for determining causation in medicine. A famous example is the discovery of the bacterium *H. pylori* as the cause of gastritis and peptic ulcers during an era when ulcers were thought to be caused by stress (a popular villain for many diseases), suppressed anger, or spicy food. In the early 1980s Australian pathologist Robin Warren and Australian physician Barry Marshall finally succeeded in culturing the bacteria from the stomach (by accident, actually; they had unintentionally left their petri dishes incubating for five days over a holiday weekend). Their paper arguing that *H. pylori* was the culprit, forget anger and Thai food, initially met with resistance and skepticism, but within a few years other researchers verified the association of the bacteria with gastritis and ulcers. Then, to demonstrate that *H. pylori* was the cause and that the association was not merely coincidental, Marshall offered up his body to science. He drank a beaker of *H. pylori* culture and within a few days became ill with nausea and vomiting. Subsequent tests confirmed signs of gastritis and the presence of *H. pylori*. Marshall and Warren went on to demonstrate that antibiotics are effective in the treatment of many cases of gastritis and ulcers. Their work was recognized with a Nobel Prize.

The causal chain is only as strong as its weakest link, and disproving a single item of evidence can overthrow the entire hypothesis. That is why Koch's postulates function best in the field of microbiology. You can't apply them in the field of epidemiology, the arena, as science writer Gary Taubes explained, where most controversies about causation in health and disease take place.[69] Epidemiologists try to identify patterns and correlations across studies of different and often enormous populations, and their conclusions rest on whatever statistical associations emerge. But as statisticians and college teachers forever try to impress on students and laypeople, *correlation does not imply causation.* Two things may be statistically correlated but in reality have nothing to do with each other. The number of storks nesting in certain European villages is reportedly correlated with the number of babies born in those villages, but (as far as we know) storks don't bring babies, and babies don't attract storks. It's just that human births are more frequent at certain times of year, and those peaks happen to coincide with the storks' nesting periods.

Storks and babies are an example of an illusory correlation, an apparent association between two things that is merely coincidental. Illusory correlations can cause great personal and social suffering as well as social harm. Claims of an association between autism and vaccination for childhood diseases alarmed many parents, but study after study has failed to find any connection whatsoever. In one definitive study of all children born in Denmark between 1991 and 1998 (over half a million children), the incidence of autism in vaccinated children was a bit lower than in unvaccinated children. The apparent link between vaccination and autism is almost certainly a coincidence, an illusory correlation, arising from the fact that symptoms of childhood autism are often first recognized at about the same time that children get a series of vaccines.[70]

Because of the problem of illusory correlations — as well as the statistical likelihood that in a sample of many thousands of people, some correlations will occur just by chance — epidemiological evidence in determining the cause of a disease cannot be as scientifically rigorous as Koch's postulates. Epidemiological studies form a *mosaic* of scattered findings rather than a linked chain. Unlike with a chain, which can be broken by one weak link, cutting out one piece of a mosaic may weaken the overall picture but it will not destroy it. Contradictory findings simply alter the balance of probability that a hypothesis is correct.[71]

By understanding the mosaic created by epidemiological studies, we can see why so many medical hypotheses persist long after they have been disconfirmed and why so many studies in health and medicine keep contradicting one another — to public exasperation. Well, *should* I get B_{12} injections? Well, *is* coffee harmful? Once you told me that margarine was healthier than butter and now you tell me that butter is better. Well, which is it?*

---

* Only if you are seriously deficient in vitamin B_{12}. Coffee is fine. Butter is better.

It is true that on rare occasions, correlational evidence may be strong enough to support causation. In 1775, a British surgeon with the wonderful name of Percivall Pott noticed a marked rise in cases of scrotal cancer in his clinic, almost invariably in young chimney sweeps. When two rare events strongly intersect, the association between them implies causality. And, indeed, chimney sweeping and scrotal cancer were both uncommon enough that the overlap between the two stood out starkly, and Pott could safely infer that chimney sweeping increased the risk of scrotal cancer. Eventually, that inference was scientifically confirmed, and Pott became the first scientist to demonstrate that a cancer may be caused by an environmental carcinogen. Such a convincing association between rare events, however, is the exception.

How, then, should we approach the mosaic of findings that occur with more complicated diseases, such as breast cancer?

The Physician as Detective

Austin Bradford Hill, the British biostatistician who pioneered the randomized clinical trial in the 1940s, offered an answer. He suggested that a case for causation in epidemiology, unlike in microbiology, should be structured in the same way a detective proves a case: the preponderance of pieces of evidence, rather than a single definitive experiment, establishes cause.[72] In 1965, he proposed nine "viewpoints" (which came to be referred to as the Bradford Hill criteria) that he suggested could help scientists determine whether there is a causal relationship between the proposed agent and the specific disease. Let's look at the eight most relevant to our story.

Strength: The evidence must be strong; that is, statistically significant and not trivially so.

Consistency: The evidence must be consistent across different studies and populations.

Specificity: When a risk factor or cause produces a specific result, it adds support for the hypothesis. In epidemiology, it is often difficult to achieve such specificity, because the spread and incidence of a disease is frequently a result of many factors, but the absence of specificity supports the inference that A is not the cause of B.

Temporal relationship: Exposure to the risk factor always precedes the outcome.

Dose-response relationship: An increased dose of or exposure to the risk factor should lead to increased incidence of the disease, and, conversely, the incidence of the disease should decline when exposure to the factor is reduced or eliminated.

Plausibility: The evidence and the theory behind it must be plausible, agreeing with the currently accepted understanding of the disease-causing processes. A chance correlation, as between shoe size and flute-playing ability, is implausible.

Coherence: The association between factor A and disease B should be compatible with existing knowledge. Of course, a new theory and supporting data can overturn an orthodox assumption and cause a paradigm shift. But if a hypothesis or belief—say, that the world was created six thousand years ago or that giraffes can levitate— requires a major sacrifice of everything known about archaeology, physics, biology, and anthropology, that theory is likely to be invalid.

Experiment: The disease can be prevented or ameliorated by a particular experimental intervention.

Finally, we want to add a ninth criterion: consideration of *alternative explanations,* which is a fundamental ingredient of the scientific method. Before concluding that A causes B or that A increases the risk of B, scientists must consider other possible explanations of B and rule them out.

The relationship between cigarette smoking and lung cancer is a good example of a convincing mosaic of evidence. The causal relationship meets all of Hill's criteria:

Strength: The data show a 1,000 to 3,000 percent increase in the risk of lung cancer in smokers compared to nonsmokers.

Consistency: The strong association between cigarette smoking and lung cancer has been confirmed in almost all studies.

Specificity: Eighty-five percent of all lung cancer patients are or were smokers. Some lung cancer patients, although nonsmokers, were exposed to secondhand smoke, a possible risk factor for the disease.

Temporal relationship: The practice of smoking precedes development of the disease, apart from the minority of cases in which the nonsmoking patient had a genetic predisposition or exposure to other carcinogens.

Dose-response relationship: The more cigarettes that people smoke and the more years they smoke, the greater their risk of lung cancer.

Plausibility: Cigarette smoke has been shown to cause pre-malignant changes in the lungs of laboratory animals. Similar changes have been seen in the lungs of smokers, including those who later developed lung cancer.

Coherence: The association between smoking and lung cancer conforms to existing physiological research and theory.

Experiment: As rates of smoking and exposure to second-hand smoke have declined, so have rates of lung cancer. Conversely, as rates of smoking rose among women, so did rates of lung cancer.

Alternative explanations: Other risk factors in lung cancer have been ruled out or understood to apply in only a minority of cases.

Now, using Hill's framework, is the link between oestrogen and breast cancer supported?

Strength: The link is unsupported. Most of the correlations published by the WHI and other investigators were neither strong nor statistically significant by conventional standards.

Consistency: The link is unsupported. Most studies find no consistently increased risk of breast cancer associated with oestrogen alone. On the contrary, the results could not be more inconsistent: Between 1975 and 2000, 45 studies examined the relationship between breast cancer and oestrogen. In 82 percent of these, no increased risk; in 13 percent, a very small increased risk; and in 5 percent, a decreased risk. In that same 25-year period, of 20 studies of HRT, 80 percent found no increased risk, 10 percent found an increased risk, and 10 percent found a decreased risk.[73]

Specificity: The link is unsupported. The overwhelming majority of breast cancer patients have never taken oestrogen, and the vast majority of women who have taken hormones have never developed breast cancer.

Temporal relationship: The link is unsupported. Taking oestrogen does not always, or even frequently, precede the onset of the disease. The risk of breast cancer increases with age—even after menopause, when oestrogen declines, and even among women who never took oestrogen.[74]

Dose-response relationship: The link is unsupported. Study after study finds no consistent increased risk of breast cancer in women who have taken oestrogen or HRT for five years, ten years, or fifteen years. If cumulative exposure to oestrogen is a risk factor in breast cancer, why did the Nurses' Health Study and the Million Women Study find that tiny risk only among current users rather than past users? Some investigators assert that early menarche and late menopause, which would provide a woman with more exposure to oestrogen in her lifetime, are associated with an increased risk of breast cancer. But, as we saw, they are not.

Plausibility: The link is unsupported. Surely, the strongest disconfirming evidence for the claim that oestrogen causes breast cancer is this: the administration of oestrogen has been shown to have beneficial effects even in women with advanced breast cancer. One of the first physicians to discover this was Sir Alexander Haddow, director of the Institute for Cancer Research at the University of London, who in 1944 reported that 25 percent of his patients with advanced breast cancer improved when given high-dose oestrogen.[75]

Researchers in the United States and around the world have gotten the same or better results. Oncologist Bruno Massidda and his team in Italy reported remission in 50 percent of advanced breast cancer patients treated with oestrogens,[76] and so did Reshma Mahtani and colleagues at the Boca Raton Comprehensive Cancer Center.[77] Gabriel N. Hortobagyi and colleagues at the MD Anderson Cancer Center reported that the most effective therapy for metastatic carcinoma of the breast was combined oestrogen-progestin.[78] James Ingle and colleagues at the Mayo Clinic demonstrated better survival among breast cancer patients treated with diethylstilbestrol (DES), a form of oestrogen, compared to tamoxifen,[79] as did Per Eystein Lønning and colleagues in Norway.[80] And the pioneer cancer researcher V. Craig Jordan and his research team demonstrated that both high and low doses of oestrogen can shrink cancerous breast tumors.[81]

Coherence: The link is unsupported. Using the mosaic method of knowledge, the more pieces we add, the clearer the overall image should become. That is what happened in confirming the relationship between smoking and lung cancer, and it is precisely what has *not* happened in the persistent efforts to confirm a relationship between oestrogen and breast cancer.

Experiment: The link is unsupported. The largest randomized experiment to determine a link between oestrogen and breast cancer, the WHI's study, failed to do so. The withdrawal hypothesis—that women who went off HRT when the study was halted were less likely to develop breast cancer—did not hold up. And the WHI also showed that oestrogen alone is actually associated with a decreased risk of breast cancer and breast cancer death.

Alternative explanations: Not ruled out. When researchers fail to confirm their hypothesized link between risk factor A and disease B, they are then supposed to consider other explanations and explore other risk factors. But over and over in the studies of oestrogen and breast cancer, we see researchers unable to accept their own evidence of small, weak, contradictory, or nonexistent links. Instead of considering alternative explanations, they have often resorted to data mining or retrospective substratification to try to find *something,* somewhere in the data that supports their belief that a significant association must be in there.

The simplistic effort to make oestrogen the bad guy ignores the remarkable complexity of human cells and of cancer itself. V. Craig Jordan, who discovered that tamoxifen could prevent breast cancer, has a highly creative alternative explanation of oestrogen's contradictory effects. He postulated that collections of malignant cells, like other living organisms, must adapt to their environment in order to survive. Thus, certain breast cancer cells, which seem to depend on oestrogen to proliferate, will die when oestrogen is removed from their environment—which supports the "Don't give breast cancer survivors oestrogen" position. But with the passage of time, these same malignant cells become immune to the effects of oestrogen deprivation and then die when oestrogen is reintroduced into their environment—which explains why Jordan and others have effectively used oestrogen to shrink breast cancers.

Bradford Hill ended his 1965 paper by saying, "All scientific work is incomplete—whether it be observational or experimental. All scientific work is liable to be upset or modified by advancing knowledge. That does not confer upon us a freedom to ignore the knowledge we already have, or to postpone the action that it appears to demand at a given time."

The Take-Home

In summary, the hypothesis that oestrogen is a real risk factor in breast cancer fails to meet Austin Bradford Hill's criteria. Why, then, has the belief that oestrogen causes breast cancer persisted? Because fear sells.

The tobacco industry fought the data showing a link between tobacco and lung cancer with a powerful weapon: doubt. An unpublished tobacco industry report drawn up in 1969 stated their strategy explicitly: "Doubt is our product, since it is the best means of competing with the body of fact."[82] But anti-smoking advocates had their own weapon, something just as visceral: fear—and fear of the most terrifying illness, cancer. Today, the reports linking

HRT to breast cancer rely on fear rather than doubt to fortify their arguments, perhaps because doubt does not generate as much attention or emotion. But the fear of HRT is misplaced. After all, the percentage of lung cancer patients who were smokers is approximately 85 percent, and the current cure rate for lung cancer is approximately 15 percent.[83] By contrast, the percentage of breast cancer patients who have ever used HRT is 11 to 24 percent, and the 2021 cure rate for newly diagnosed breast cancer patients is 90 percent; for women with localized breast cancer, which is the stage found in the majority of newly diagnosed cases, the five-year survival rate is 98 percent.[84]

But fear sells, which is why, whenever someone manages to assemble yet another huge vat of numbers and pull out a small but spurious "finding" that can alarm women, headlines follow like a dog after a biscuit. In 2019, the *Lancet* published a paper claiming that HRT increases the risk of breast cancer, generating the inevitable media attention, and so we scrutinized the study closely. Once again, the data did not support the alarm.[85] In 2023, a Danish study immediately generated unnecessary anxiety about a possible connection between HRT and cognitive decline. That is not remotely what the study found, as we will show in chapter 6.

The irony is that as early as 2007, some of the senior WHI investigators were trying to distance themselves from the fears they had aroused in so many women. When interviewed for a *Scientific American* article that year, Jacques Rossouw said, "My surmise is that women just got scared of hormonal therapy across the board, irrespective of what they were using it for." (Never mind that it was he and his colleagues who scared them with "across the board" claims of risk.) He added, "With hindsight you could say, well, maybe we should have emphasized reasonable use even more." (Well, yes, you sure should have.) The study's abrupt halt also stoked fears. Maybe we didn't need to terminate the study so abruptly, admitted WHI investigator Marcia Stefanick. "It wasn't an emergency—it wasn't like people were, you know, under serious threat of the adverse outcomes." (But that was precisely what you told women—that they were under serious threat of breast cancer, stroke, and dementia.) "I wish we had figured out a way to change prescribing practices but have fewer people distressed about it." (How about forgoing that scary and exaggerated press conference then?) Senior investigator JoAnn Manson said, "Taking all of the previous research into account"—which is precisely what the WHI did not do—"there may have been a reason to look very closely at differences by age and differences by time since menopause. Had that been part of the earliest reports, it might have helped put the results into perspective for younger women." (Yes, it would have, and she, at least, has publicly modified her position over the years.[86])

All worthy comments, followed by silence. No press conferences recanting previous statements. No public retractions. On the contrary, the WHI continued its campaign of fear throughout the first decade of the 2000s and after. In 2008 they reported that among the women who had received HRT, even years after they stopped taking it, the death rate from all causes was "somewhat higher than among those assigned to placebo"—even though this difference in mortality, once again, did not reach statistical significance. This nonsignificant increase in mortality, they added, "was accounted for by deaths attributed to various cancers unrelated to the pre-specified trial outcomes... most prominently lung cancer."[87]

What? No increased mortality from breast cancer, and suddenly we are talking about lung cancer? Not to worry; they quickly dropped that concern.

Notice, by the way, that phrase "cancers unrelated to the pre-specified trial outcomes." Researchers don't get to go back into their data and predict *new* "trial outcomes" after the fact. At least the WHI didn't try to relate breast cancer risk to astrological signs.

When the WHI investigators failed to get strong and clear results, they often opted to speak of "trends" in their data that "suggested" risk and then seemed to experience amnesia when those "trends" went away. In 2003, they reported that HRT increased the risk of ovarian cancer.[88] When challenged on the fact that they offered no statistically significant data to support that claim (then or subsequently), they responded that HRT "may increase" the risk of ovarian cancer, reminding us smugly that "these data arose from the only randomized, double-blind, placebo-controlled trial." Sorry, folks. It doesn't matter how big, fancy, and costly your study is if it does not yield reliable results.

Undeterred, in 2009 Chlebowski and colleagues claimed that women randomized to HRT had an increased risk of dying from lung cancer.[89] This assertion was, as usual, based on retrospective substratification, which might be why they reported an increased risk of lung cancer *deaths,* not of lung cancer *incidence.* (How is that possible? HRT will kill you before it even makes you sick?) They ominously warned that "postmenopausal women, especially those at elevated baseline risk of lung cancer, such as current smokers or long term past smokers, should consider this additional hazard before beginning, or continuing, combined menopausal hormone therapy." They neglected to cite other studies that reported a *reduced* risk of lung cancer associated with postmenopausal hormone therapy[90] as well as a *reduced* risk of lung cancer deaths among women taking either oestrogen alone or HRT.[91] Raising a concern about lung cancer in the context of limited and conflicting data is misleading and potentially harmful. And, by the way, the WHI has not said another word about lung cancer since then.

*　　*　　*

The National Cancer Institute biostatistician Robert Hoover once told his colleagues: "The scientific method I was taught involved setting a hypothesis and then trying everything you could to destroy it, and if you couldn't, then you began to accept it. Somehow we've gotten away from that. We develop hypotheses and then we do everything we can to find something that supports it."[92] That's not the way we should be doing science. Although we agree with Henry James's witty admission that "nothing is my last word on anything," we do think it is time to relegate the "common knowledge" that oestrogen causes breast cancer to the dustbin of discredited ideas—along with the theories that radical mastectomy is the best treatment for primary breast cancer, that anger causes peptic ulcers, and that stress causes tuberculosis.

3

Can Breast Cancer Survivors Take Oestrogen?

Dear Dr. Bluming:

My wife survived breast cancer ten years ago, and since then she has suffered from strong symptoms of perimenopause. So strong, in fact, that three years ago the doctors were testing her to rule out ALS for her fatigue, muscle weakness, and muscle tingling, which she still lives with. We have strived to do our homework as thoroughly as possible, yet our long search for a doctor willing to even consider a short span of HRT (to at least prove the cause of the symptoms) has led nowhere. After our most recent rejection, I wrote to the doctor afterward: "I wonder if perhaps it's been me all along who has been grossly misunderstanding the experts I've been reading and listening to. So, I did a quick search and found a link to Oestrogen Matters, *which disputes those experts. What am I missing here? What does the science actually tell us? And more important, why is it that my spouse is being denied the agency to weigh for herself the pros and cons of HRT treatment based on currently available probabilities?"*

Thus far, we have been addressing concerns that many healthy women have: Will taking hormones increase the risk of breast cancer? Will they alleviate menopausal symptoms? In this chapter, Avrum will make a counterintuitive but well-supported claim that even among women who have had breast cancer, HRT is a reasonable option for those suffering from severe menopausal symptoms. It's Av's story, so he will tell it from his point of view.

*   *   *

Several years ago, I was called to be an expert witness for the prosecution in a medical malpractice case involving a patient with lung cancer. The diagnosis had been delayed for over a year because the radiologist had missed an abnormality on the patient's chest X-ray. The tumor, which could have been surgically removed a year earlier, was now inoperable.

I clearly remember being cross-examined by the attorney for the defense. He held up a large, weighty textbook, *Cancer: Principles and Practice of Oncology,* and asked: "Dr. Bluming, isn't it true that this textbook is called the bible of cancer medicine?" I told him I was thoroughly familiar with the textbook, which was highly respected in my field, but that no book of medicine is a bible. He handed it to me and asked me to open it to a particular page and read a marked paragraph about lung cancer. The paragraph asserted that since the prognosis in lung cancer was invariably fatal, early diagnosis was of no benefit to the patient. The attorney asked for my response. "There is a reference in this paragraph to a specific article," I said, "which, by a fortunate coincidence, I have brought to the trial." I read the article for the court. It stated that early diagnosis and treatment in that type of lung cancer would greatly improve the chance for cure. The textbook author had misquoted the article. The cancer bible was fallible.

I haven't been that lucky with any specific reference since, one that clarifies an issue and its resolution in one shot. On the contrary, I am well aware that in the practice of medicine, physicians can invariably find references to support almost any opinion. I have attended many medical conferences that degenerated into an exercise of dueling references, with each side citing only those articles that supported its position. That is why I have made every effort to seek not only the studies that support my opinions but also the studies that contest them. When you are a physician, the question of the evidence you rely on to make a decision about an intervention or treatment becomes more than an academic debate at a conference or in a journal; your patients' well-being, health, and often lives depend on the advice you offer and the decisions you make. You therefore want the very best evidence to guide your practice, while also leaving room for your years of experience and clinical judgment.

Yet sometimes there isn't a good reference to guide you; sometimes there are no clear answers. In my lifetime in oncology — and I became an oncologist before the specialty was even named — two clinical decisions were of paramount personal importance to me: whether or not to endorse the movement away from radical mastectomy in favor of the less invasive lumpectomy and whether or not to prescribe HRT for patients whom I had treated for breast cancer.

In the mid-1970s, I moved from an academic appointment in Boston to the private practice of medical oncology in Southern California. At that time, several clinical investigators around the world were exploring lumpectomy followed by radiotherapy as an alternative to traditional mastectomy for the treatment of newly diagnosed breast cancer. This was a dramatic departure from standard medical practice, and many surgeons reacted with understandable resistance. "The only way to reduce the risk of recurrence is to remove the breast and as much adjacent tissue as possible," many said, "and now you are telling me to remove only the lump? Anything less than total mastectomy would be malpractice." At my hospital, the chief of surgery would go from operating room to operating room asking the surgeons what surgery they were performing. When the surgeon replied, "A mastectomy," he would shout, "Way to go!"

My fellow Los Angeles oncologists strongly advised me not to pursue the issue of lumpectomy and not to recommend it to my patients. I would be dependent on surgical referrals to help build my practice, they said, and mastectomy was bread-and-butter surgery for practicing surgeons. By trying to alter the paradigm of how breast cancer should be treated, I would turn off referrals from these necessary sources. Since all of my medical training had been done back east, I had no hospital or university contacts that might supplement patient referrals to my new oncology practice. I thanked my new colleagues, but I did not follow their advice. I decided on a plan of cooperation and persuasion instead of an adversarial battle.

As chair of the professional educational committee of the

American Cancer Society for the San Fernando Valley chapter, then the second largest in the nation, I invited Sam Hellman, a professor and chair of the department of radiation therapy at Harvard Medical School and one of the early pioneers of lumpectomy research, to speak to a large audience of physicians and surgeons. His data were powerful and persuasive, and I could see that the edges of the iceberg of doubt and opposition in that room were melting. But it took the surgeons' own experiences to fully persuade them. Mike Drickman, one of the first surgeons in Los Angeles to switch to lumpectomy, told me that after he did his first one, "I was so overwhelmed by the gratitude of the patient that whenever I can, I offer lumpectomy as the first option to all my breast cancer patients who need surgery."

To further my collaborative approach, I invited physicians across specialties to begin a community-wide study in which they would assemble data on their patients and then chart what happened after lumpectomy. The community team consisted of eight medical oncologists, seventeen breast surgeons, seven radiation therapists, and seven pathologists, and when I wrote up the results of our study for the *Annals of Surgery*, I listed all 39 of us as co-authors. The editor, who must have been amused by all those names marching across the page, told me I could have only three. But I was grateful for, and proud of, my colleagues for their open-minded yet critical review of emerging data in this field, so I replied that I wanted all of those names not only printed but also identified by specialty. By this, I hoped to recognize their willingness to work across different areas of expertise, highlight the diversity of perspectives they brought to the research, and encourage further community collaborations of this kind. The editor agreed.[1] Referrals to my practice did not suffer, and the Los Angeles community became one of the earliest adopters of this new treatment for primary breast cancer.

As a physician, I rely on the medical literature to inform me of what the empirical evidence shows, but I also depend on other physicians' clinical experience. The greatest challenge in the practice of oncology is finding the best approach to a medical problem at the time you need it, even when that approach might not yet have been published. Many years ago, I was asked to see a 16-year-old boy with newly diagnosed Ewing's sarcoma of a rib. At that time, the cure rate for this disease was close to zero. His grandmother ignored this information and said to me, "Dr. Bluming, I did not survive Auschwitz to watch my grandson die of cancer."

I reviewed the world literature and learned that no treatment had been successful. I consulted Mark Nesbitt, chair of the National Ewing's Cooperative Group, who had no therapeutic suggestions. I consulted Gus Higgins, the principal investigator of the children's Cancer Study Group in Los Angeles; he didn't have any promising leads either. I consulted Audrey Evans, a leading medical oncologist at Children's Hospital in Philadelphia; she did have a protocol for treatment but little evidence of its success. I eventually found Gerald Rosen, a pediatric oncologist at Memorial Sloan Kettering Cancer Center in New York. He had treated more than 50 young patients with Ewing's sarcoma using a combination of intensive chemotherapy drugs, and he was having remarkable success. In the overwhelming majority of his patients, he told me, the cancer had disappeared and not returned, even after several years. He had not yet published the results of his intensive regimen; it would be another year before he did. But I was persuaded by the fact that he had more experience with this rare tumor than anyone else, and he was getting encouraging results. I used his regimen with my patient. That was more than thirty years ago, and that teenager is now a healthy middle-aged man.

The practice of oncology thus requires a constant dance between what we know and what we must learn; perhaps that's why we say that surgeons *perform* surgery but physicians *practice* medicine.

In the early 1990s, my wife and many of my other breast cancer patients began asking me if they could take HRT. For women who have survived breast cancer, chemotherapy typically induces menopause and intensifies its symptoms.[2] Dawn Hershman, leader of the Breast Cancer Program at Columbia University, reported that women treated with chemotherapy, compared to those who had no chemo, were 5.7 times more likely to report vaginal dryness, 5.5 times more likely to report painful sexual intercourse, 3 times more likely to report decreased libido, and 7.1 times more likely to report difficulty achieving orgasm.[3] Between 66 and 96 percent of breast cancer survivors report having severe hot flushes, night sweats, and insomnia, and the great majority fail to receive treatment for these annoying and uncomfortable symptoms.[4] Most cancer survivors are understandably preoccupied with coping with the effects of their illness and relieved that its treatment is over. No wonder they are therefore inclined to endure menopausal symptoms as an inevitable side effect of chemotherapy.

And yet, over time, many of my patients yearned for relief from the severe menopause-associated symptoms that were impairing the quality of their lives. I was understandably apprehensive. So were they. It seemed a no-brainer. Why would I even consider administering oestrogen to women with a history of breast cancer? What if the cancer returned? What if I were responsible for the death of a patient who, without my well-intentioned help, might have remained cured? I felt pangs of empathy for the surgeons who could not give up doing radical mastectomies, unable to shake the fear that it would put their patients at greater risk of recurrence. Nonetheless, the frequent requests from my patients for something to alleviate their distress motivated me to seek new answers.

STEP ONE: LOOKING FOR CLUES

In those days, we didn't have enough good data on the consequences of giving HRT to breast cancer survivors for oncologists to say for sure that it was harmful, beneficial, or neither. Like the experts I consulted for Ewing's sarcoma, physicians who were doing the best they could with limited research to guide them, some oncologists were prescribing hormones for their breast cancer patients, but they did so with varying degrees of follow-up and no consistent treatment protocol.

So I had to look for clues in related conditions. Where might I see whether oestrogen increased the risk of recurrence in women who had had breast cancer? I started by evaluating the then-common belief that premenopausal breast cancer survivors should have their ovaries removed as a precaution. Because the ovaries produce oestrogen, and because oestrogen was "known" to cause breast cancer, that intervention made sense. But it was wrong. William Creasman, a gynecologic oncologist, observed that prospective randomized studies showed that removing a woman's ovaries had no benefit in reducing the risk of recurrence of cancer or in prolonging a woman's survival, which is why it is no longer done (though, as with all procedures in medicine, there are a few diehards who still believe it is beneficial). "Thus, oestrogen appears to be all right in the premenopausal breast cancer patient," he wrote, "but, for some reason, oestrogen administration to the postmenopausal patient is not. Why?"[5]

Next, because oestrogen and progesterone levels soar during pregnancy, I looked at what research had to say about women who become pregnant after having breast cancer. Alan Wile, a surgeon, and Philip DiSaia, chair of the division of gynecologic oncology, both at the University of California, Irvine, had just reported that pregnancy, either during or after treatment for breast cancer, had no negative effect on prognosis. They also noted that there was no benefit in removing their patients' ovaries and that as long as patients were informed "that there is no evidence that oestrogen has an adverse effect upon established breast cancer," they felt it was appropriate to let them take HRT to alleviate menopausal symptoms and improve well-being.[6]

Thus far, I was finding that neither lowering oestrogen levels (by removing ovaries) nor raising oestrogen levels (becoming pregnant) increased the recurrence of breast cancer. And I kept finding the considerable historical evidence of oestrogen's benefits. In 1966, Charles Huggins was awarded the Nobel Prize for showing that hormones could control the spread of some cancers. He gave a sample of rats a carcinogen that produced breast cancer and then administered high levels of estradiol and progesterone for thirty days. The hormones inhibited the emergence of breast cancers and only one week of treatment was enough to demonstrate this effect.[7]

It took years before Huggins's Nobel Prize–worthy findings were applied to women, but the results were promising. I noted with interest three studies conducted in the 1980s by researchers in Europe and England:

—Torben Palshof, an oncologist in Copenhagen, and his colleagues reported on 332 patients with breast cancer who, after surgery and radiation, were randomly assigned to be given either DES (diethylstilbestrol, a form of oestrogen), tamoxifen, or placebo for two years. Five years later, the women receiving DES had the lowest rate of cancer recurrence, similar to the rate of women given tamoxifen, and the women on the placebo had a significantly higher recurrence rate. The lowest recurrence rate (zero) was seen among women who had ER+ tumors and were given DES. When Palshof conducted another follow-up in 1985, the results were unchanged.[8]

—Louk V.A.M. Beex, an oncologist in the Netherlands, and his colleagues randomized 63 postmenopausal women with advanced breast cancer to receive tamoxifen or oestrogen to see how their tumors responded. Although tamoxifen was believed to block oestrogen and therefore be more beneficial, both were equally effective: the tumors in 33 percent of the patients on tamoxifen shrank, and so did those of 31 percent of patients on oestrogen.[9]

—Basil Stoll, a British endocrinologist who wrote an early textbook on hormonal management in patients with breast cancer, reported that he had administered oestrogen and progesterone to 65 postmenopausal women with advanced breast cancer. After six months of treatment, 22 percent of the women showed a regression of the cancer.[10]

I also discovered numerous oncologists who were risking the disagreement and even outright opprobrium of colleagues by saying that the time was right for research on giving HRT to breast cancer survivors. For example, Michael Baum, who was then chair of the Breast Cancer Trials Coordinating Committee in London and a member of the academic department of surgery at the Royal

Marsden Hospital, wrote, "I find it intolerable that we should have to carry on in ignorance about the benefits and risks of prescribing hormone replacement therapy to women who have had breast cancer. There are occasions when the indications for hormone replacement therapy must take precedence over any theoretical objections. It is clearly inhumane when a woman who is already having to cope with the physical and psychological burden of breast cancer is then expected to accept, without relief, some of the serious effects of the menopause, which can include severe depression."[11]

With this empirical and clinical grounding, I felt ready to launch a study in which HRT would be administered to breast cancer survivors who were in complete remission following treatment but who were suffering from menopausal symptoms affecting the quality of their lives. They would be followed over time to see if HRT increased the risk of the breast cancer's return.[12]

STEP TWO: DEALING WITH THE FDA

I began by discussing my research proposal with most of the medical oncologists in the Los Angeles area as well as with gynecologists and primary-care physicians. Their participation was crucial in giving me critical evaluations of the data I would be collecting and the assumptions I was making. Many of them added their own patients to the study once it was under way. All supported going ahead with the study, but several expressed one major reservation: a fear of legal culpability if a woman in the study had a recurrence. I therefore contacted Ned Good, the president of the California Bar Association, who told me that anybody can sue anybody for anything, and we would have no guaranteed protection from a lawsuit. However, he added, the best proactive defense would be to ensure that every patient understood the risks entailed in joining the study and to have that understanding confirmed with a signed informed-consent form. Done.

I then called the Food and Drug Administration, told them what I was planning to do, and asked whether I needed FDA approval to proceed. They said that if I called what I was doing a *treatment*, FDA approval was unnecessary; some physicians, they were aware, were already administering HRT to breast cancer survivors without FDA approval. If, however, I wished to call what I was proposing a *study*, then I was advised to submit a full protocol to the FDA, with details of the methods, goals, rationale, and references from the medical literature. That took a little longer, but I did it.

Six weeks after receiving my proposal, a doctor at the FDA called to tell me that it had been put on a clinical hold, primarily because the FDA felt that the study would place women at an increased risk of breast cancer recurrence.

"Has anyone there actually read my full proposal?" I asked him. "The part where I describe the studies indicating that oestrogen is safer than most physicians realize, even for breast cancer survivors?"

"Don't shoot me," he said. "I'm just the messenger."

I asked to speak to someone who had decision-making ability, and, instead of having a second phone conversation, I was invited to testify before an FDA subcommittee in Rockville, Maryland, on February 14, 1992. Before leaving, I met with Alan Wile, one of the breast cancer investigators who I knew had called for such research. We rehearsed a joint presentation. I offered to coordinate a pilot study for three hundred women, and Alan, speaking for his department at UC Irvine, agreed that if we found no increased risk of breast cancer recurrence in the pilot study, his university would commit to a long-term, double-blind, randomized study of this issue with a population of five thousand postmenopausal women.

We delivered our presentations at the committee meeting, which was open to the public. One women's health activist implored the panel to deny our proposal, arguing that giving oestrogen to women who had had breast cancer was tantamount to giving them a "poison valentine." But at the end of the meeting, Barbara Hulka, a prominent epidemiologist who was chair of the committee, said she thought it would be unethical *not* to do this study. On the flight home, Alan cautioned me not to think our study had been approved.

"It sounded like approval to me," I said.

"Just wait," he advised.

Several weeks later, the FDA let us know that although they had approved the study in principle, they objected to the details I had specified for a small pilot study. The only proposal they would approve, they said, would be for a prospective double-blind randomized trial of six thousand to eight thousand women. I protested this decision because, as the committee members were aware, some breast cancer survivors were already being treated with HRT in pockets around the country, with no attempt to collect relevant data. We would be collecting follow-up data on our treated patients rather than allowing their results to be lost. If we were harming them, surely, we felt, it would be preferable to discover this in a small pilot study rather than a large one.

"Sorry," the FDA said (in effect). "The big study or none."

Undeterred, I returned to the FDA on my own dime, and, to its credit, the FDA organized another committee meeting to hear me out. Before the formal discussion began, some of the physicians on the committee asked me questions that felt surreal.

"Why don't you do a different study?" one male doctor asked. "Why are you fixated on doing this particular one?"

"I *do* other studies," I said. "However, because the evidence persuades me that we have been wrong about oestrogen's harms, and because we don't know enough about giving oestrogen to breast cancer survivors, I feel this study is important."

"Why do you even need to do this study?" asked a female physician. "Isn't it true that most of your patients are going to die anyway?"

"I'm sorry, but you are misinformed," I told her. "The current cure rate for early breast cancer is now running higher than 85 percent."*

"Perhaps I should refresh my knowledge on the subject," she said.

"That would be good," I agreed.

During the several-hour committee meeting that followed, I was unable to convince any member that the pilot study I proposed was worth doing before undertaking a larger study of several thousand women. As I was leaving, I asked the chair what would happen if I returned to my community and proceeded with the study I wanted to do. "We can't tell you how to practice medicine, Dr. Bluming," he said. "I hope you have found our comments to be beneficial." I thanked them for taking the time to meet with me but told them I found their comments to be of no help. I returned to Los Angeles to run the study.

Step Three: Doing the Pilot Study

At least the FDA had unanimously concurred that my proposed research was ethical. "We agree," they (eventually) wrote in *JAMA*,

---

* Today the cure rate percentage, as noted in chapter 2, is in the 90s.

"that clinical trials are needed to address this issue [of HRT for breast cancer patients] and wish to note that on February 14, 1992, the Division of Metabolism and Endocrine Drug Products of the FDA convened its Fertility and Maternal Health Drugs Advisory Committee for public discussion of the issues involved. During the proceedings, the committee voted unanimously yes to the question: is it ethical to conduct well-designed clinical trials of hormone replacement therapy in women who have been treated for breast cancer, when a primary outcome of interest will be to ascertain whether the treatment causes breast cancer recurrence?"[13]

As soon as I returned home, I addressed the annual meeting of the Los Angeles Obstetrical and Gynecological Society and officially launched the pilot study of the effects of hormone replacement on breast cancer survivors. I made sure that every woman understood the potential benefits and risks of the medication, as well as the purpose of the study. And I made sure that the "caution statement" from the FDA was clearly positioned in the informed-consent form:

Although the FDA has endorsed the rationale for testing the potential benefits and risks of hormone replacement therapy in women with a history of treated breast cancer, the FDA committee responsible for reviewing this particular study feels that no meaningful data will be provided due to the small number of patients to be evaluated (300) and the absence of a randomized group of comparable women who will receive no hormone replacement therapy. The FDA committee raised the concern that any results from so small a study population on non-randomized patients might be overinterpreted to yield conclusions of benefit or risk that were premature or inaccurate.

All of the women gave their consent. Because I knew that a symptomatic woman would know whether or not she was receiving oestrogen within a few days—after all, these women wanted to take HRT precisely to alleviate menopausal symptoms—there was no placebo control group. (The problem of keeping participants from knowing whether they are getting the real drug or a placebo afflicts much research, even the august Women's Health Initiative.) I did, however, compare the hormone-treated group with women who had been diagnosed with the same stage of breast cancer, who had been treated the same way over the same period, and who lived in the same community. If I were to discover an unanticipated risk of recurrence among my patients or find any research demonstrating an increased risk—that is, any evidence that giving my patients HRT was pouring fuel on a fire—I would halt the study immediately.

I began this work in 1992, and for the next fourteen years I published an annual update on the participants, with 100 percent follow-up on the 248 women who were enrolled over time. Even the women who had moved out of state during those years provided me with medical information on how they were doing.[14] My goal was to determine whether these women showed an increased incidence of recurrence of breast cancer in the same breast, developed cancer in the other breast, or developed breast cancer metastases elsewhere in the body.

And this is what I found: they did not. Yes, a few of these women had a recurrence of breast cancer, but not at a rate higher than the comparable women who were not on HRT.

In 1997, I was invited to present the five-year results of our study to 8,500 oncologists at the annual conference of the American Society of Clinical Oncology (ASCO) in Denver. The presentation preceding mine was given by a physician from the National Cancer Institute. He told the crowd that "the NCI is not sponsoring HRT symptom relief or disease prevention studies in breast cancer survivors." Based on the computer models, he concluded, "Hormone replacement therapy can only harm breast cancer survivors."

I remember thinking I would probably be stoned for presenting my small pilot study from a community in Southern California after this preemptive condemnation by a spokesperson from the National Cancer Institute. But that's not the way it turned out. After my presentation, all the questions and comments from this large, international audience of leading oncologists and researchers were positive. In contrast, the audience's response to the NCI presentation was uniformly negative.

"Don't shoot me," the NCI guy said. "I'm only the messenger."

The following year, 1998, the FDA informed me that the clinical hold that had been placed on my study six years earlier — the study I had continued, reported on annually, and presented at the 1997 ASCO annual meeting — was being lifted.

This response from ASCO and the FDA was, of course, gratifying. But it was even more gratifying to realize that my study was now part of a larger phenomenon: the medical establishment's resistance to treating breast cancer patients with HRT was melting, just as its resistance to lumpectomy had melted a decade before. In a thorough review of the research up to 1994, Melody Cobleigh, a medical oncologist, and her colleagues in the Eastern Cooperative

Oncology Group noted that the main concern about prescribing oestrogen for women who have had breast cancer is that "dormant tumor cells might be activated. There is surprisingly little clinical information to substantiate such concern."[15]

By then I was used to oncologists and epidemiologists finding "surprisingly little clinical information" to support the prohibition of HRT for breast cancer survivors. In 2000, Henk Verheul, a medical oncologist at the Cancer Center of Amsterdam, and his associates wrote that none of the current treatments for breast cancer—surgery, radiation, chemotherapy—were negatively affected by oestrogen, even oestrogens that were administered at concentrations that are *considerably higher* than those in typical prescriptions of HRT. The available studies, they concluded, "fail to demonstrate that, once breast cancer has been diagnosed, oestrogens worsen prognosis, accelerate the course of the disease, reduce survival or interfere with the management of breast cancer. It may therefore be concluded that the prevalent opinion that oestrogens and oestrogen treatment are deleterious for breast cancer needs to be revisited."[16]

In Finland, gynecological researchers Olavi Ylikorkala and Merja Metsä-Heikkilä observed that because the number of women surviving breast cancer has been increasing steadily, health professionals need to face the issue of how best to treat their symptoms of menopause and improve their health in general. (Ylikorkala's own research had documented the benefits of HRT in reducing the risk of vascular dementia and heart attacks in postmenopausal women.) The "categorical refusal [to prescribe HRT] is a double-edged sword because it also denies these women all the undisputable health benefits HRT provides," they said. "This refusal is not however supported by the observational data available so far on this question, because HRT has not increased the risk for breast cancer recurrence."[17]

Throughout the 1990s, wanting to make sure that my own study's findings were not outliers, I kept track of any studies conducted anywhere in the world that compared breast cancer survivors given HRT with matched controls. None were the huge RCT trials of thousands of women that the FDA hoped someone would do someday. Some had small samples, some had larger ones; the length of time women were on HRT varied considerably; some followed up on their patients for a few months or two years or five years or longer. But if you are prepared for another boring litany of good news, here it is:

- Slovenia: Oncologists Marjetka Uršič-Vrščaj and Sonja Bebar compared 21 women with breast cancer who were treated with HRT for an average of 28 months with two controls for each patient. Result: No increased recurrence of breast cancer among the women on hormones.[18]
- Australia: There were three Australian studies. In one, John Eden, senior lecturer in reproductive endocrinology at the University of New South Wales, compared 90 breast cancer survivors treated with HRT for a median of eighteen months and followed for a median of seven years, with 180 matched controls. Result: A small but significantly reduced recurrence of breast cancer among the women on hormones.[19]
- In another, gynecologist Jennifer Dew compared 167 women with a history of breast cancer who received HRT with 1,122 women with a similar history who were not given HRT. Result: No increased recurrence of breast cancer among the women on

hormones, even among women whose tumors were oestrogen-receptor positive. Four years later, she updated her study with an even larger sample. Again, the use of HRT was not associated with an increased risk of recurrence of breast cancer.[20]

- In a third, gynecologist Eva Durna conducted a retrospective observational study of 286 breast cancer survivors given HRT compared with 686 breast cancer survivors who did not take HRT. (The women were followed for a median of under two years, but some had been on HRT for up to twenty-six years.) Result: Significantly lower rates of recurrence and rates of death from breast cancer in women who used HRT compared with nonusers. Two years later, she reported a second study of 524 women who were diagnosed with breast cancer when they were still premenopausal. Of the 277 who reached menopause following their diagnosis and treatment, 119 took HRT to control symptoms. The risks of recurrence of or death from breast cancer were no different among those women who took HRT and those who did not.[21]

- France: Oncologist Marc Espie followed 120 patients who received HRT after treatment for breast cancer, matching each patient with two comparable controls, for 2.4 years. Result: No increased recurrence of breast cancer among the women on hormones.[22]

- Finland: Merja Marttunen and colleagues reported on 131 breast cancer survivors, 88 of whom decided to take oestrogen and 43 of whom chose not to. All were followed for a mean of 2.6 years. Result: No increased recurrence of breast cancer among the women who chose oestrogen.[23]

- Germany: Matthias Beckmann and colleagues at the Friedrich Alexander University in Erlangen retrospectively reviewed the records of 185 breast cancer patients, 64 of whom took HRT and 121 of whom did not. Result: Even after five years, no increased recurrence of breast cancer among the women on hormones.[24]

Across the United States, researchers were coming to the same conclusion:

- Houston, Texas: Rena Vassilopoulou-Sellin, at the MD Anderson Cancer Center, conducted a randomized prospective study in which 39 breast cancer survivors were treated with Premarin and compared to 319 similar patients who did not receive hormones. Result: After four years, no increased recurrence of breast cancer among the women on HRT.[25]
- Irvine, California: Gynecologic oncologists Wendy Brewster and Philip DiSaia matched 125 breast cancer patients who were taking oestrogen alone or HRT with 362 breast cancer patients who received no hormones. Result: No increased recurrence of breast cancer among the women on hormones.[26]
- Troy, Michigan: Medical oncologist David Decker conducted a prospective study of 277 breast cancer survivors who received oestrogen for a mean duration of 3.7 years, matched with comparable controls. Result: No increased recurrence of breast cancer among the women on hormones.[27]
- Dallas, Texas: George Peters, professor of surgery, compared 64 breast cancer survivors treated with oestrogen after their diagnosis with 563 breast cancer survivors who were not.

Result: After an average follow-up of 12 years, no increased recurrence of breast cancer among the women on hormones.[28]

- Seattle, Washington: Cancer researcher Ellen O'Meara reviewed the records of 2,755 women, ages 35 to 74, who had been diagnosed with breast cancer between 1977 and 1999. Of those, 174 women were taking HRT after treatment. Each was matched with four control women identified from the same cohort over the same period and followed for a median of 3.7 years. "HRT after breast cancer has no adverse impact on recurrence and mortality," she concluded. Instead, HRT users had significantly lower breast cancer recurrence rates, breast cancer mortality rates, and overall mortality rates compared to nonusers.[29]

- Milwaukee, Wisconsin: Linda N. Meurer and Sarah Lená conducted a review of nine independent observational studies and one randomized controlled trial. Result: Breast cancer survivors using HRT had no increased risk of recurrence compared with controls. In their meta-analysis — totaling 717 women who used HRT after being diagnosed with breast cancer compared with 2,545 women who did not — the survivors who were taking oestrogen had significantly fewer deaths (3 percent) over the study periods than the women who were not (11.4 percent).[30]

Right now you might be saying, "Wait! What about all the studies that found an increased risk of recurrence?" I thought you'd never ask. There weren't any. Until the Women's Health Initiative, this time with an ally: the HABITS study.

THE OPPOSITION WEIGHS IN

When the WHI announced its findings in 2002, the first major consequence was that millions of women who had been taking HRT discontinued it within the year.[31] But three other events occurred almost immediately as well. First, research on hormones halted; of the 18 studies that began in the 1990s in which survivors of breast and other cancers were being treated with HRT, virtually all of them stopped dead in their tracks. Mine was the only one to continue recruiting patients and gathering data.

Second, the FDA added a black box warning to the label of Prempro (Wyeth's version of HRT), and this dire caution remains today on all preparations of oestrogen:

WARNINGS: CARDIOVASCULAR DISORDERS, BREAST CANCER, ENDOMETRIAL CANCER AND PROBABLE DEMENTIA.

Pretty scary. The label also cautions that patients should take the smallest dose of hormones for the shortest time possible—an admonition, as we will see, that is not supported by evidence.

And third, thousands of lawsuits were filed almost immediately. A lawyer who represented Wyeth told me that at the height of litigation, Wyeth (and Pfizer, which had bought Wyeth) faced more than ten thousand lawsuits. About eight thousand cases in federal court were centralized in Arkansas, in a legal procedure that speeds the handling of complex liability suits. The others were spread out in state courts around the country. Of the dozens of trials, the results were mixed; the defense won some, and the plaintiffs won others. The largest plaintiffs' settlement was $78.74 million. "In a 2012 securities filing, Pfizer reported that it paid $896 million to resolve about 60 percent of the cases," the lawyer wrote. "The mass media, not good science, drove the litigation and the decisions of women with regard to their postmenopausal healthcare."[32]

Well, you say, of course an attorney representing Wyeth would complain that "the mass media, not good science, drove the litigation." But many oncologists, gynecologists, and researchers agree with that statement. "I have become somewhat frustrated since the WHI report," my late colleague Phil DiSaia, at UC Irvine, wrote to me. "The media are not interested in facts. They seem to be focused on sensationalism. The fact that oestrogen therapy alone carried no increase in the incidence of breast cancer was placed on page 18 in a small paragraph. Whereas, the borderline statistics on hormone replacement therapy was front-page news."[33]

DiSaia was especially disheartened by the paralyzing effect that the WHI had had on his own research. He had "become convinced that hormone replacement therapy is *not* contraindicated in breast cancer survivors and does *not* increase incidence of recurrence," and therefore he had been trying to launch a prospective, randomized study through the gynecologic oncology group at his medical school—the very study that the FDA had wanted done. "On each occasion the medical oncologists in the Group voted it down," he said, because of the WHI. At the time, they had nearly two thousand patients registered and ready for the study to begin.

The WHI was not the only punch. A second blow landed in 2004 with the publication of the HABITS study (an awkward acronym formed from the study's name: Hormonal Replacement Therapy After Breast Cancer—Is It Safe?). The WHI investigators immediately took the results to be a confirmation of their view that hormones were harmful in general and even more so for women who had had breast cancer. Rowan Chlebowski, whom you met in the previous chapter, wrote in an editorial about the HABITS study that it "may arguably not be the definitive word on the use of hormone therapy in women with breast cancer but it will probably be the last word when considered in context of our evolving under-standing of the effects of hormone therapy on chronic disease in women."[34] Not the definitive word but the last word? What does that mean?

I read the HABITS report announcing the termination of the study with great interest. It appeared to contradict everything I've been telling you, and it is still the most widely referenced study dealing with HRT for breast cancer survivors. The study, led by Lars Holmberg at the University Hospital's Regional Oncologic Center in Uppsala, Sweden, proposed to randomize 1,300 breast cancer survivors to HRT or no HRT and follow them for five years. The end point was the development of any new breast cancer: a recurrence in the original breast, a new lesion in the other breast, or a distant metastasis.

The study was prematurely terminated in 2003 after only two years of follow-up and after only 434 women of the proposed 1,300 had been enrolled. The reason for the sudden termination was the disproportionate number of women on HRT who developed another breast cancer: 26 women in the HRT group (20 percent) and only 7 in the non-HRT group (4 percent). Those numbers—26 versus 7—seemed striking and important.[35] Few observers noticed that the groups did not differ in their incidence of metastatic disease or risk of death during that time, and when Premarin was used as the source of oestrogen, there was no increased risk of breast cancer either.

The investigators updated their results in 2008 with follow-up on more participants.[36] The results were still concerning: this time, 39 women in the HRT group (17.6 percent) and 17 in the non-HRT group (7.7 percent) had developed new breast cancers. It is primarily on the basis of this difference between 39 and 17, a total of 22 women, that HRT is being denied to millions of breast cancer survivors around the world.

Should it be? Maybe not. HABITS had serious limitations: It found no new breast cancers among women who had had positive lymph-node involvement (which is believed to increase the risk of recurrence), no difference between groups in the incidence of distant metastases, no differences in the risk of deaths from breast cancer, and no new breast cancers in women taking oestrogen alone. And this time, the increased risk for women on HRT turned up only among those who were also taking tamoxifen. Now, this was very odd because tamoxifen causes a dramatic increase in circulating oestrogen levels in premenopausal women, but this does not impair its therapeutic benefit. Even the HABITS study's lead investigator, Lars Holmberg, noted: "We agree that the results of a single randomized study should be interpreted cautiously, especially when the study is terminated early. We reported why we stopped recruitment in the HABITS trial and have not claimed to say 'the final word.'"[37]

Around the same time as the HABITS trial was being conducted, another study of Swedish breast cancer survivors, the

Stockholm study, was under way. It was also a prospective randomized trial, similar in size to HABITS. Yet this study, in which 188 women were randomized to receive HRT and 190 got none, found no difference in the development of new breast cancers among HRT users as compared to nonusers. And also like the HABITS trial, it found no difference in mortality between the two groups. After 10 years, these findings were unchanged.[38]

Critics and professional societies weighed in on the HABITS study almost immediately. William Creasman, whose research I previously described, noted some troubling problems: More than 20 percent of the women were not included in the analysis because they had not had at least one follow-up visit. The choice of hormone regimen — Premarin or other combinations of oestrogen and progesterone — was left to the treating physician, so there was no uniformity in what was prescribed. Anomalies across the randomized groups were overlooked; 11 women who were supposed to be taking HRT were not, and 43 women who were not supposed to be taking HRT were. Important risk factors in breast cancer are its stage and the status of lymph nodes, but this information was not provided at the time the women were randomized to get hormones or not. Further, baseline mammograms were not mandated. Why does this matter? You're a breast cancer survivor who has entered the study to see if hormones will increase or decrease your risk of recurrence. But the investigators don't give you a mammogram first to see if there is any evidence of a local cancer. The importance of this omission is crucial, since the only increased recurrences noted were local. Were the risk factors for recurrence the same in the two groups? We don't know.

Creasman was especially annoyed by the editorial commentary

that accompanied the HABITS article. "This study can reasonably guide clinical practice of women with breast cancer," the editorial had concluded. The hell it can, Creasman said, in essence, although he used the measured tones of medical writing: "This conclusion seems premature and without merit." He was unaware of any data indicating that HRT was harmful to breast cancer survivors except for the HABITS study, which contained the flaws he'd enumerated. "With the exception of the HABITS study," he wrote, "all the other data do not identify the deleterious effects of replacement therapy in the post-cancer patient. To deny such therapy for life-disturbing symptoms does not seem to be in their best interest."[39]

What "other data" was Creasman referring to? Of the 20 studies published between 1980 and 2005, *only* the HABITS study found an increase in breast cancers among women on HRT, and *only* if they were also taking tamoxifen. Alfred Mueck, head of the department of endocrinology and menopause at University Women's Hospital in Tübingen, Germany, and his colleagues agreed: a few prospective randomized studies and at least 15 observational studies that investigated HRT after breast cancer were available, they wrote, and "only the HABITS study shows an increased risk of relapse."[40]

The Society of Obstetricians and Gynaecologists of Canada was not impressed by HABITS either. In 2005, its members issued a policy statement that included these two summary points: "HRT after treatment of breast cancer has not been demonstrated to have an adverse impact on recurrence and mortality," and "HRT is an option in postmenopausal women with previously treated breast cancer."[41] But JoAnne Zujewski, head of Breast Cancer Therapeutics in the Clinical Investigation Branch at the National Cancer Institute, took the opposite view. "Combined with the negative results of the WHI, most U.S. physicians and their patients have gotten the message that long-term HRT can be harmful. The things they were trying to treat with hormone replacement therapy we now have better measures for," she said, "such as bisphosphonates for the prevention of osteoporosis and aspirin or statins for cardiac health."[42] This acceptance of faulty data for both the presumed harms of HRT and the alleged benefits of its alternatives—and without a discussion of the side effects, harms, and lack of efficacy of those alternatives—is, to my mind, reprehensible.

Where do matters stand today? When you have many studies pointing in one direction, and one renegade study that points the other way, you have to ask: What was wrong with all of the preceding studies, or why did this anomaly turn out as it did?

Long after HABITS, in a review of observational and randomized studies of breast cancer survivors titled "Use of Hormone Therapy for Menopausal Symptoms and Quality of Life in Breast Cancer Survivors: Safe and Ethical?," two gynecologists answered that question with an unqualified yes.[43] In 2022, I did my own review of the 25 (now 26) available studies in which HRT was given to breast cancer survivors.[44] You can see the results of the 26 studies in Table 1: Six reported reduced risk of recurrence; 4 reported reduced mortality from breast cancer; the rest found neither an increased nor decreased risk. Of the 5 studies in which women were randomly assigned to take HRT or not, 4 reported no increased risk of breast cancer. Only one, the HABITS trial, reported an increased risk.

Table 1. Summary of the 26 Studies of
Breast Cancer Survivors Given HRT*

Year published	No. on HRT/No. of controls	Results
1. 1980	37/95 Prospective randomized	**Reduced recurrence**
1a. 1985 follow-up	51/103	**Reduced recurrence** **Reduced mortality**
2. 1988	14	No recurrences
3. 1993	35	2 recurrences in 35 No breast cancer deaths
4. 1995	90/811	**Reduced recurrence**
5. 1997	43	1 recurrence in 43 No breast cancer deaths
6. 1998	167/1305	No difference
7. 1999	120/240	No difference
8. 1999	20	No recurrences
9. 1999	50/26	No difference
10. 1999	21/42	No difference
11. 1999	39/280	No difference
12. 2000	125/362	**Reduced mortality**
13. 2000	51/49 Prospective randomized	No difference
14. 2001	56/551	No difference
15. 2001	88/43	No difference
16. 2001	64/121	No difference
17. 2011	174/698	**Reduced recurrence** **Reduced mortality**

18.	2002	56/243 Prospective randomized	No difference
19.	2002	286/836	**Reduced recurrence** **Reduced mortality**
20.	2003	277/554	No difference
21.	2003	230	No difference
22.	2004 and 2008	174/171 and 221/221 HABITS study and follow-up: Prospective randomized	**Increased risk of** **local tumor or in** **opposite breast;** **no increased risk** **of metastasis or** **death**
23.	2005 and 2013	175/184 and 188/190 Stockholm study and follow-up: Prospective randomized	No difference
24.	2008	117/63	**Reduced recurrence**
25.	2008	708/1399	No difference
26.	2022	133/6371	No difference (all women ER+)

* For a full list of references, see Bluming AZ, "Hormone replacement therapy after breast cancer: It is time." *Cancer J* 2022;28:183–90, and *J Natl Cancer Inst* 2022;114:1347–54.

By now you should not be surprised that even excellent researchers who are blinded by the paradigm that "breast cancer survivors must not take oestrogen" would be convinced that HABITS was the final word. They literally do not see the data in front of their eyes.

Over the years, various investigators did their own reviews (meta-analyses) of the studies that were available. I looked carefully at the existing 20 reviews published between 1994 and 2021. In all of them, only HABITS supported the claim of an increased risk of breast cancer among survivors. None of the reviewers were skeptical of HABITS's limitations, and several, convinced of HRT's harm, misinterpreted and exaggerated the data from other studies as well.

For example, in one meta-analysis done in 2005, Nananda Col and her coauthors, one of whom was Rowan Chlebowski, commented on "the sharp increase in risk [of breast cancer recurrence] observed even after short-term HT use in randomized trials," and they noted that "the increase in risk pertained to distant as well as local recurrences."[45] Wrong on two counts. First, HABITS found no increased risk of distant recurrences. Second, *sharp* increase? This claim rested on one case-control study by Ellen O'Meara. We have already noted O'Meara's unequivocal bottom line, but if you missed it earlier, here it is: "HRT after breast cancer had no adverse impact on recurrence and mortality." O'Meara found "lower risks of recurrence and mortality in women who used HRT after breast cancer diagnosis than in women who did not."[46]

Consider a 2020 review article concluding that HRT is "disadvantageous and thus contraindicated" in breast cancer survivors.[47] Tamás Deli and his coauthors incorrectly reported that the Stockholm trial found that HRT users had an increased risk of breast cancer recurrence compared with nonusers. But it didn't. The Stockholm report clearly stated that "after 10.8 years of follow-up, there was no difference in new breast cancer events" and "there was no overall risk for breast cancer recurrence." Deli's team went on to assert, also incorrectly, that the HABITS and Stockholm studies found "increased mortality" associated with length of time women were on HRT. Flat wrong. The HABITS trial concluded that "there was no convincing evidence for a higher breast cancer mortality associated with HT exposure" and the Stockholm trial reported "no increased mortality from breast cancer or other causes from HRT."

Similarly, in a 2022 review of four RCTs, Francesca Poggio and her team concluded that the use of HRT to mitigate symptoms "may be associated with an increased risk of disease recurrence in these patients."[48] To reach this misleading conclusion, they focused on the two studies that claimed to find recurrences. One, of course, was HABITS. The other investigated not oestrogen but tibolone, a compound that is not available in the United States and that has no reported oestrogenic effect on breast tissue or the endometrium.

And so HABITS was not the definitive, or even the last, word after all. Far from providing a clear answer, it gave WHI supporters like Rowan Chlebowski and JoAnne Zujewski the chance to "see" the dangers of HRT, and it gave people like William Creasman, Phil DiSaia, and me the chance to "see" the many flaws in that conclusion.

*   *   *

Five years after the Women's Health Initiative study appeared, two of its supporters presented their data at the annual San Antonio Breast Cancer Symposium. Afterward, I debated them on a radio program in front of a studio audience. Our debate was cordial, but it was clear to me that both men regarded my position with contempt.

"You'll find, Dr. Bluming," said one, an internationally respected biostatistician, "that statistics aren't everything."

"You should know," I replied. "You're the statistician."

During a break, he looked away from me and said loudly, so that everyone in the room could hear, "I believe that administering

HRT to women with a history of breast cancer is malpractice." Remembering the surgeons who once thought it was malpractice to perform lumpectomies, all of the studies except HABITS that supported my position, and the gratitude of the many women in my own study, I could only offer to continue the debate.

Where are we today? While most new research stopped after the WHI, investigators have continued to reassess existing evidence with meta-analyses. Pelin Batur, an internist affiliated with the Cleveland Clinic, and her colleagues reviewed 15 studies totaling 1,416 breast cancer survivors using hormone replacement therapy compared with a cumulative control group of 1,998 patients.[49] The majority of the women began HRT between two and five years after their diagnosis, and they remained on it for an average of three years. Compared to nonusers, the women on HRT had a 10 percent decreased chance of recurrence and even a slightly reduced mortality rate from cancer or other causes. Using the most recent data from the National Cancer Institute on rates of cancer incidence and survival in the United States, Batur calculated that the 7-year cancer-related mortality rate for invasive breast cancer was 17.9 percent for nonusers and 4.5 percent for the women on HRT.

The Take-Home

Years ago, Melody Cobleigh and the Cooperative Oncology Group suggested a new guideline for the practice of medicine. Treating breast cancer survivors with oestrogen had been hindered, they argued, by the physician's maxim *Primum non nocere* ("First, do no harm"). "Such moralizing prevents moral reflection," they wrote. "The task of moral reflection is to assess whether something is right or wrong." Given the lack of evidence that oestrogen is detrimental to breast cancer survivors and given its potential positive effects, they proposed a new medical maxim: *Primum certior fi, tunc mone* ("First understand, then advise").[50]

In 2023, Eric Winer, president of the American Society of Clinical Oncology, exhorted his fellow physicians to realize that partnering with patients is crucial for clinical care and beneficial research. "Now, more than ever before, we need to reach out to our own patients," he said, "to understand what we need to prioritize to make their lives better, and we need to listen to their guidance."[51] This has been my philosophy and practice in all my career, and it extends to my own family.

When my daughter, Ariel, was 35, she discovered a tumor in her breast that turned out to be cancer. Because her mother, Martha, had been diagnosed at 45, a fairly young age too, Martha underwent testing to see if she might have passed on a genetic predisposition to breast cancer. All the tests were negative. Ariel had the tumor removed and received follow-up radiation. She had been unable to conceive even before the diagnosis, and eventually she had in vitro fertilization, which produced a healthy daughter.

Twelve years later, when Ariel entered perimenopause, she asked me whether she should start HRT. We spoke at length and she read an early draft of this book. "Dad, I'm confused," she said. "Until now, whenever I needed advice on a medical course of action, you pointed me in the direction you felt was right. There was never any problem with your advice. So why won't you just tell me whether or not you think I should start HRT?"

I told her what I would tell any reader of this book. "I cannot guarantee the cancer will not come back," I said, "with or without

HRT. I want you to remain healthy through what I hope will be a long life to come, and I've provided you with the evidence of HRT's benefits and risks. Both you and I recognize that a decision not to take HRT has consequences—you would lose its many benefits—just as the decision to take it does."

I thought of the wise observation of Siddhartha Mukherjee: "It's easy to make perfect decisions with perfect information," he wrote in *The Laws of Medicine*. "Medicine asks you to make perfect decisions with imperfect information."[52]

On my advice, but with her full understanding, Ariel decided to take HRT.

4

Matters of the Heart

Dear Dr. Bluming:

My gynecologist is against oestrogen not because of breast cancer risk, but because of the increased risk of heart disease. She thinks that statins are much safer than hormones and she is really pushing them on me to lower my cholesterol, even though I've never had heart problems. Is she right on this?

Although breast cancer is the most common cancer affecting women in this country, lung cancer kills more women than breast cancer does, and both pale next to heart disease, which is the leading cause of death in American women. In 2021, one of every five female deaths was caused by heart disease — that's 310,661 women — compared to the 43,600 women who died from breast cancer that year. And recall that amazing statistic in chapter 2: Of the many thousands of women who develop some form of breast cancer, approximately 90 percent are disease-free after five years, and for women whose initial breast cancer was localized—which is the vast majority of cases—98 percent are disease-free after five years.[1] In spite of these reassuring statistics, breast cancer generates more anxiety than heart disease.

Many women fear breast cancer more than heart disease because they believe breast cancer kills more women than heart disease, starting at a younger age. However, that belief is wrong: In every decade over age 40, more women die of heart disease than breast cancer. Surprising, isn't it? This has been the case for decades. The National Council on Aging commissioned a survey of 1,000 women between the ages of 45 and 64, finding that "61% said that the disease they most feared was cancer—predominantly breast cancer. By contrast, only 9% said that the condition they most feared was the disease most likely to kill them—heart disease."[2]

In spite of its unmistakable risk to women, heart disease remains almost invisible to them. Women often say to us, "But I know so many women who have had breast cancer, and so few who have had heart problems!" One reason may be, as we now know, that symptoms of heart disease, congestive heart failure, and heart attacks in women often differ from those in men; the familiar heart-attack symptom of crushing pain in the chest and left arm is more common in men than women, and the primary signs in women are usually unrelated to chest pain. (They include discomfort in the neck, jaw, shoulder, upper back, or stomach, shortness of breath, pain in one or both arms, nausea, sweating, dizziness, and extreme or unusual fatigue, all of which can indicate many different problems.) Unlike in men, atherosclerotic disease in women may be hard to confirm. Many women who go to their doctors or the ER with symptoms of acute coronary syndrome have angiograms that are normal, demonstrating no obstructive coronary artery disease.[3] Indeed, in 2019, one-third of women who died of a sudden cardiac arrest had had normal ECGs.[4]

New York internist Marianne Legato established the Foundation for Gender-Specific Medicine precisely because of the evidence showing that the results of studies based on white men did not invariably apply to women or other ethnicities, and heart disease was one area in particular where the sexes differed. In her 1991 book *The Female Heart,* Legato touted the benefits of oestrogen in reducing the risks of heart disease. A decade later, in *Women Are Not Small Men,* Nieca Goldberg, medical director of NYU's Center for Women's Health, also described the different ways that the sexes experience heart disease.[5] It is a message that cardiologists have been trying to convey ever since, though it is often drowned out in the pink-ribbon campaigns about breast cancer. (The American Heart Association has valiantly promoted its own campaign, Go Red for Women.)

Another reason that women underestimate the risk of death from heart disease may stem from what cognitive psychologists call the availability heuristic, people's tendency to judge the probability of an event by how easy it is to think of instances of it and how emotionally compelling those instances are. Catastrophes and shocking accidents evoke a strong emotional reaction and thus stand out in our minds, becoming more available mentally than other negative events. This is why people overestimate the frequency of deaths from tornadoes and underestimate the frequency of deaths from asthma, even though the latter occurs dozens of times more often than the former. It is also why women overestimate the frequency of deaths from breast cancer and underestimate the frequency of deaths from heart disease. Years ago, people in Europe and America were in a panic about mad cow disease, which affects the brain and can be contracted by eating meat from contaminated cows, and several French researchers did a creative field study to see how reporting affected public fears. Whenever newspaper articles reported the dangers of mad cow disease, beef consumption fell the following month. But when news articles reported the same dangers using the technical names of the disease—Creutzfeldt-Jakob disease and bovine spongiform encephalopathy—beef consumption stayed the same.[6] The more vivid label caused people to react emotionally and overestimate the danger. During the entire period of the supposed crisis, only six people in France were diagnosed with the disease, but an image of a mad cow—that sweet, placid creature running amok—is highly available.

In the same way, breast cancer is more available mentally than heart disease. Indeed, people are so attuned to the politics and fundraising efforts surrounding breast cancer that when a female celebrity is diagnosed with it she often goes public—as did Christina Applegate, Kathy Bates, Judy Blume, Diahann Carroll, Sheryl Crow, Julia Louis-Dreyfus, Melissa Etheridge, Edie Falco, Olivia Newton-John, Cynthia Nixon, and Tig Notaro. Most women have heard the 1-in-8 statistic for the incidence of breast cancer in women by age 85, but most people are unaware that the incidence of prostate cancer is comparable. For example, in 2018, there were 287,850 cases of female breast cancer with 43,250 deaths, and 268,490 cases of prostate cancer with 34,500 deaths. Yet the public hears much less often about the equally famous men who have had the disease—including Harry Belafonte, Jerry Brown, Robert De Niro, Rudy Giuliani, Ian McKellen, Michael Milken, Roger Moore, Mandy Patinkin, Colin Powell, and Ben Stiller.

Although never diagnosed with breast cancer herself, Angelina Jolie released the news that she had the BRCA gene, an inherited genetic predisposition to develop breast cancer, and had chosen to have a double mastectomy. Revelations like Jolie's are seen as brave acts to raise public awareness, which of course they are and they do, and they evoke enormous sympathy and support. Yet when a female celebrity announces that she has a cardiovascular issue, she doesn't get the love and teddy bears. Miley Cyrus did write in her memoir about having an intermittently elevated heart rate (tachycardia), which is not life-threatening, and Rosie O'Donnell blogged about her heart attack, but they are rare. Heart disease remains a leading but invisible killer. We suspect that grieving fans of Carrie Fisher and June Carter Cash took little note that Fisher died of cardiac arrest and Carter died of complications from heart surgery.

Even women who have had breast cancer are more likely to die from heart disease than from breast cancer. Epidemiologist Jennifer Patnaik and her colleagues studied a population of 63,566 women diagnosed with breast cancer at the age of 66 or older, following them for an average of nine years. Heart disease was responsible for more deaths among this large population than breast cancer. "Attention to reducing the risk of cardiovascular disease," the researchers concluded, "should be a priority for the long-term care of women following the diagnosis and treatment of breast cancer."[7]

Today this recommendation is widely accepted among oncologists. At the 2017 San Antonio Breast Cancer Symposium, Anne

H. Blaes, a medical oncologist, described her work with SERMs (selective oestrogen-receptor modulators), nonchemotherapy drugs that are often given to postmenopausal breast cancer survivors after their primary treatment. These drugs are generally prescribed for women with no residual evidence of breast cancer and are usually administered for a minimum of five years. Because SERMs have the potential to damage cells that line the coronary arteries, Blaes cautioned that they might do more harm than good, because "most women with breast cancer are at greater risk of dying from cardiovascular disease than from breast cancer."[8] In 2018, the American Heart Association, in its first official scientific statement on cardiovascular disease and breast cancer, concurred.[9]

DOES HRT HARM THE HEART? HOW WOULD WE KNOW?

Perhaps the most obvious evidence of oestrogen's benefit for heart health is that menopause is the dividing point between *before* and *after*. Before menopause, women are protected from cardiovascular disease, relative to men, by their existing levels of endogenous oestrogen. But after menopause, women have cardiovascular disease complications that *exceed* those of men. Although heart disease increases with age in both sexes, it occurs two to six times more often among postmenopausal than premenopausal women across the age range of 40 to 54. Because the risk of heart disease rises so sharply after menopause,[10] many studies have sought to determine whether the increase is due to normal aging (the rates rise in men too, after all) or to the drop in oestrogen. Is oestrogen providing those significant cardiovascular benefits for premenopausal women? Compelling evidence suggests that it is.

Elizabeth Barrett-Connor, who until her death was principal investigator of the Postmenopausal Oestrogen/Progestin Interventions trial (PEPI), and epidemiologist Trudy Bush reviewed the existing studies and concluded that "most, but not all, studies of hormone replacement therapy in postmenopausal women show around a 50% reduction in the risk of a coronary event in women using unopposed oral oestrogen."[11] In their own study of nearly 900 women, they found that oestrogen plus progestin was actually better than oestrogen alone in reducing the risk of heart attacks. Francine Grodstein, a lead investigator on the Nurses' Health Study, reported that oestrogen reduced the development of primary cardiovascular disease by nearly 40 percent.[12] And in two separate studies, women who'd had their ovaries removed had an increased risk of coronary artery disease, but that risk was minimized if they took oestrogen.[13]

Some scientific investigators have quarreled with the validity of these studies, which are among the most respected observational studies in the medical literature, precisely because they are observational and not randomized controlled trials (RCTs). That is why we want to take a moment to explain their concerns and where we think they're wrong.

As we have noted, RCTs are considered the ideal method of conducting medical research; in an RCT, women are randomly assigned to receive hormones (or any other treatment whose effectiveness is being tested) or a placebo, and, when the study is double-blind, neither they nor the investigators know who is taking what.

However, observational studies have several advantages over randomized controlled trials: they are less expensive, can be done more quickly, can include a broader range of patients, and can be conducted when an RCT would be impossible or unethical. In observational studies, participants are not randomly assigned to a treatment group or a control group; they are simply observed over time to see whether the intervention helped, harmed, or did nothing, compared with a similar group who received a placebo or no treatment at all. The main problem with this method is that if women can *choose* whether or not to take hormones instead of being randomly assigned to hormones or a placebo, the women who choose to take it may be different in ways that influence the outcome. Perhaps healthier, more educated women choose to take hormones, and it's their health and education that are responsible for any health benefits, not the medication.

In the 1970s and 1980s, researchers who were comparing RCTs with observational studies identified another problem: earlier observational studies tended to inflate positive treatment effects. One analysis showed that more than half of the observational trials of a particular treatment concluded that it was effective, but only 30 percent of the double-blind, randomized controlled trials did.[14] Understandably, many researchers decided that observational studies should not be used at all for evidence-based medical care. "If you find that [a] study was not randomized," said the authors of a 1997 book on evidence-based medicine, "we'd suggest that you stop reading it and go on to the next article."[15]

If that were so, you'd have to stop reading this book now, because you would be wary of the observational studies we have cited, notably in the previous chapter on HRT for survivors of breast cancer. Yet, while RCTs get respect, they are not without pitfalls. Some have their own biases and statistical distortions — the Women's Health Initiative being the largest and most unfortunate example — and carefully conducted observational studies and randomized controlled trials usually produce similar results.[16] The table listing the 26 studies in which breast cancer survivors were given HRT (pages 124–25) illustrates that convergence, though only five were RCTs.

According to an in-depth review of this issue by physicians Kjell Benson and Arthur Hartz, older comparisons of the two approaches were based on studies conducted in the 1960s and 1970s, and research methods have improved since then. Observational studies conducted between 1985 and 1998, Benson and Hartz noted, were "methodologically superior to earlier studies... [including] a more sophisticated choice of data sets and better statistical methods" that might have eliminated some systematic bias. They compared RCTs and observational studies for nineteen varied medical treatments and found that "the effects of treatment in observational studies and in randomized controlled trials were similar in most areas."[17] And when other researchers scoured leading medical journals to see which medical practices had stood the test of time, comparing findings from both methods twenty years after their publication, the conclusions were still valid in 87 percent of nonrandomized observational studies and in 85 percent of randomized trials.[18]

Even Sir Austin Bradford Hill, the distinguished medical statistician and epidemiologist at Britain's Medical Research Council — the man who developed and promoted the randomized controlled trial in medicine — came to believe it had all gone too far. "Two decades after introducing the randomized controlled trial," wrote psychiatrist David Healy, "having spent years waiting for the pendulum to swing from the personal experience of physicians to some consideration of evidence on a large scale, Austin Bradford Hill suggested that if such trials ever became the only method of assessing treatments, not only would the pendulum have swung too far, it would have come off its hook."[19]

*   *   *

So let's take a look now at the WHI's claims about hormones' effects on heart disease. In 2002, the year that the WHI announced its first results, its lead investigator, cardiologist Jacques Rossouw, and his colleagues reported that women on HRT, but not those on oestrogen alone, had a slightly increased relative risk of "heart events," including angina, indications for bypass surgery or angioplasty, and death due to heart disease.[20] But when Leon Speroff, former chair of obstetrics and gynecology at the Oregon Health and Science University School of Medicine, independently reanalyzed the WHI data, he found that the increased risk of cardiac events was seen only among women who were twenty or more years beyond menopause when they joined the study.[21]

In 2007, Rossouw and his fellow investigators revised their findings, now concluding that women who started HRT within ten years of the onset of menopause actually *reduced* their risk of coronary artery disease, while those who started after that slightly increased their risk.[22] The Nurses' Health Study came to the same conclusion.[23] Randomized controlled trials have likewise demonstrated that oestrogen reduces heart disease. A meta-analysis of 23 RCTs with a total of 39,049 women found a 30 percent decreased incidence of heart attacks and cardiac deaths among young postmenopausal women treated with oestrogen alone or HRT.[24] In a separate RCT, a Danish team randomized 1,006 healthy, recently postmenopausal women to receive oestrogen alone (if they had had hysterectomies), HRT, or nothing. At the ten-year follow-up, those who were taking either form of hormones had a 50 percent reduction in the incidence of acute cardiac events without any associated increase in the risk of cancer, venous thrombosis, or stroke.[25]

The reason for the WHI's contradictory findings about hormones and heart disease is almost certainly that the study was not based, as they claimed, on a sample of healthy women in their late forties and early fifties who were just entering menopause. On the contrary, as we have noted, not only was the median age of the women in their sample 63, but fully 70 percent were seriously overweight and half were obese. Nearly 50 percent were either current or past cigarette smokers and more than 35 percent had been treated for high blood pressure—major risk factors for cardiovascular disease. Only 10 percent of the women were between 50 and 54 years old, and 70 percent were 60 to 79, an age range where we would expect to find previously formed atherosclerotic plaques. This means that atherosclerosis was probably present in the WHI population when the study began, yet women with these well-established risk factors for heart disease *were not excluded* from the analysis of the effects of hormones on the heart.[26]

The WHI investigators have repeatedly stated that all of the women they recruited were healthy and that in fact good health was a prerequisite for participation. But these assertions are difficult to reconcile with the medical histories of so many of their participants. Two ob-gyn researchers who noted that "strong basic science and clinical observational evidence show a benefit of menopausal [hormone therapy] in the cardiovascular and central nervous systems" were highly critical of the WHI's "rush to generalize" from their older, at-risk sample to "all women and all menopausal HT regimens."[27] Such overgeneralization, they said, was clearly unwarranted.

In light of the studies demonstrating a beneficial effect of hormones among women with no indication of heart disease, some researchers have wondered whether hormones would benefit women with already narrowed coronary arteries and proven evidence of heart disease. In 1998, a large randomized study—the Heart and (o)Estrogen/Progestin Replacement Study (HERS)—was set up to answer that question. It found a statistically significant increase in heart events in women with known coronary artery disease prior to receiving HRT—but only during the first year of use.[28]

Why should HRT increase cardiovascular risk only in the first year of use and only among older women? Scientists have known for years that the elasticity of the coronary arteries decreases after menopause, and studies of primates (and also rats, mice, and rabbits) show that oestrogen keeps blood vessels healthy. Unfortunately, administering oestrogen after an interval of some years cannot reverse vascular damage.[29] These findings have been replicated in humans too; for example, in the (o)Estrogen Prevention of Atherosclerosis Trial (EPAT) in 2000 and the (o)Estrogen Replacement and Atherosclerosis (ERA) study in 2001.[30]

A leading explanation of the first-year-risk finding is that among women who do not have heart disease, oestrogen causes blood vessels to dilate (widen), thereby increasing the blood supply to the heart muscle. However, in women who *do* have underlying heart disease, oestrogen can potentially be harmful—it can induce inflammation in existing arterial plaques, causing a stable plaque to rupture, and it can also promote bleeding into the plaque, both of which can block critical coronary arteries. Oestrogen, with or without progesterone, may also cause platelet clumping, which can further obstruct coronary arteries. After the first year of hormone therapy, women no longer have an increased risk of cardiovascular events—even women with preexisting coronary artery disease. This analysis would explain why studies that have enrolled younger women, like the Nurses' Health Study, have found that HRT has a protective effect: Younger women are less likely to have narrowed coronary arteries or arterial plaques.

It would also explain the results of a longitudinal study of 332,202 Finnish women. During their first year after going off HRT, women had a small but statistically significant increased risk of cardiac death. Over time, the increased risk among those who stopped HRT (364 deaths) was more than double the risk for those who continued HRT (155 deaths).[31] This finding does not mean that HRT is detrimental; it suggests that when women go off HRT, the benefit to their vascular health dissipates, and their risk of heart disease becomes the same as it would have been had they never taken hormones.

This conclusion was supported in a randomized controlled trial in which 643 healthy women were divided according to time since menopause (under six years or more than ten years) and randomly assigned to receive either HRT or placebo. Every six months for an average of five years, the investigators measured the thickness of the women's carotid arteries—an indication of potential cardiovascular problems—and assessed the existence and degree of atherosclerosis with CT scans. HRT was responsible for a significantly slower progression of atherosclerosis as compared to placebo, but only when it was begun within six years of menopause. There was no benefit when it was initiated ten or more years after menopause.[32]

And so, a decade after the WHI scared women off HRT, yet another human cost of that decision emerged: an increase in coronary artery disease and death from heart disease. It was long past time for a course correction.

WHAT ABOUT THE ALTERNATIVES?

The logical question that follows from all of this research is: What should a woman do? Most physicians feel there is no reason for women to take hormones *primarily* to help forestall or prevent cardiovascular disease, given, they say, that alternatives for reducing the risk of heart disease are readily available. What are those alternatives? How effective are they?

"If you're going to use something to prevent atherosclerosis, your choice is statins, not hormones," said Jacques Rossouw, the WHI cardiologist.[33] Statins are the leading medications used to prevent atherosclerosis-related cardiac deaths in this country; they are among the most widely prescribed pills in the world. Statins such as Lipitor (which became the bestselling drug of all time in 2018) and Zocor are designed to reduce high serum cholesterol, although the level considered *high* began to drop when statins were developed, thereby creating a larger potential market. ("High" was originally 240, then 220, and then anything above 200, which produced 42 million more potential patients for the makers of statins.[34]) At first, there was so much enthusiasm about statins that physicians were advised to prescribe them for almost all patients in middle age, even those with no symptoms or history of heart disease. The excitement about the benefits of statins drowned out concerns about their side effects, which are not trivial; they include liver enzyme abnormalities, muscle weakness, joint pain, and diabetes[35] — none of which are side effects of oestrogen.

To assess the value of statins, therefore, a woman at risk of heart disease—either because she simply has a postmenopausal drop in oestrogen or because of her own risk profile (family history, smoking, obesity, and so on) — needs to know two things: Is high cholesterol on its own a significant risk factor for heart disease? And do statins, in lowering cholesterol, lower that risk? The answers are no and no.

In *The Truth About Statins,* cardiologist Barbara H. Roberts, director of the Women's Cardiac Center at the Miriam Hospital in Providence, Rhode Island, reported that statins are less effective in women than men, that they have their greatest benefit in preventing a second heart attack, and that they are more of a marketing success story than a medical one.[36] In a major review supporting that conclusion, physicians Judith Walsh and Michael Pignone analyzed 13 studies of the effects of statins on women and men with and without cardiovascular disease. The studies representing 11,435 women *without* cardiovascular disease showed that lowering cholesterol levels did not reduce overall mortality rates or lower the chances of having a nonfatal heart attack or heart disease. The studies representing 8,272 women who *already* had cardiovascular disease showed that statins did reduce the risk of nonfatal and fatal heart attacks.[37] Mario Petretta and his colleagues got the same results in their meta-analysis of 8 RCTs: statins reduced the risk of heart disease for men but not for women. (And statins did not reduce the risk of dying of a heart attack for either sex.[38])

We are telling you about these studies because the findings, especially for women, are so important and so little known. In an editorial in *JAMA* titled "Statins for Primary Prevention: The Debate Is Intense, but the Data Are Weak," Rita F. Redberg and Mitchell H. Katz sharply criticized the U.S. Preventive Services Task Force's recommendation that because statins reduce cardiovascular disease and mortality, they should be given to "adults aged 40 to 75 years without a history of CVD [cardiovascular disease] who have 1 or more CVD risk factors and a calculated 10-year CVD event risk of 10% or greater." Redberg and Katz were not persuaded. "The evidence for treating asymptomatic persons with statins," they wrote, "does not appear to merit a grade B or even a grade C recommendation."[39] Talk about an expanding market.

But here is another reason to be wary of statins: They raise the risk of diabetes. Most people are unaware of this potentially harmful consequence or dismiss it as being too rare to worry about, yet meta-analyses of statin trials show an increased risk of new-onset diabetes cases that exceed levels of risk considered acceptably "rare." In contrast, meta-analyses, including one of 107 RCTs of hormone replacement therapy, consistently find a 20 to 30 percent *decreased* risk of diabetes among women on HRT.[40] This surely is crucial information for women's health because preventing of diabetes and its associated metabolic syndrome (a cluster of conditions including elevated blood pressure and blood sugar, excess body fat around the waist, and abnormal lipid levels) is particularly important in reducing women's risk of cardiovascular disease. And for women who are not taking HRT, entering menopause increases their risk of metabolic syndrome and diabetes.[41]

Finally—and this finding always comes as a shock to people—there is no relationship between total cholesterol level and death from heart disease, especially for women. (We are not talking about subtypes of cholesterol, like LDL, or triglycerides, high levels of which are risk factors. But people tend to use the overall total as the danger sign, with 200 as the magic number to get under.) The decades-long Framingham Heart Study discovered this in the mid-1970s,[42] and there's been no modification of that finding since, but few paid any attention. Twenty years later, cardiologist and health-care researcher Harlan Krumholz, at the Yale School of Medicine, and his colleagues reported no correlation between cholesterol levels and heart disease, especially in women and men over age 70.[43] Few paid serious attention to their research either.

How about just cutting out fat, that stuff that makes us fat and clogs our arteries and causes heart disease? In *Good Calories, Bad Calories* and *The Case for Keto,* the investigative journalist Gary Taubes presented an exhaustive history of how cholesterol and fat became the leading villains in the American diet.[44] The belief that fat is the bad guy was obvious, intuitive, widely promulgated, institutionalized in medical guidelines, and eventually shown to be wrong. It's not only wrong; it's really wrong. Fat isn't always a culprit, and often it's a benefactor. Consider the fascinating 2017 findings from the Prospective Urban Rural Epidemiology (PURE) project, which followed individuals age 35 to 70 in eighteen countries for about seven years.[45] The investigators kept meticulous dietary records of all 135,335 participants and later assessed their overall mortality and major cardiovascular events (fatal cardiovascular disease, nonfatal heart attack, stroke, and heart failure). And this is what they found:

- Intake of total fat and each type of fat (saturated, monounsaturated, and polyunsaturated) was associated with a *lower* risk of total mortality.
- Higher saturated fat intake was associated with a *lower* risk of stroke.
- Total fat and saturated and unsaturated fats were not associated with risk of heart attack or death from cardiovascular disease.
- Higher carbohydrate intake was associated with a *higher* risk of total mortality.

Another huge meta-analysis of studies of nearly 350,000 participants who were followed for 5 to 23 years showed that "intake of saturated fat was not associated with an increased risk of CHD, stroke, or CVD" and "consideration of age, sex, and study quality did not change the results."[46] Ain't science full of surprises?

The Take-Home

When it comes to the issue of oestrogen and heart disease, the basic questions are these: How do the risks and benefits of hormones balance out, and what evidence should women and their physicians trust to help them make decisions?

First, as Howard Hodis, head of the Atherosclerosis Research

Unit at the University of Southern California, and his colleague Wendy J. Mack discovered in their extensive review, the findings from randomized controlled studies — *including the WHI* — and observational studies have converged: HRT, when begun by women near or in menopause and under age 60, reduces cardiovascular disease, heart attacks, *and* overall mortality. When women stop taking hormones, death rates increase, and the biggest contributor to those death rates is cardiovascular disease.[47]

Second, oestrogen may have beneficial effects on the heart for women who start taking hormones early in menopause because oestrogen promotes healthy blood vessels and may help delay the formation of plaque. But it probably has no protective effect on women who begin using hormones in their mid-sixties and they might even be potentially risky for them, at least for the first year, if they have preexisting artery disease.

Third, statins and aspirin do not have the beneficial effects that HRT does. They have not been shown to significantly reduce women's risks of coronary artery disease and a first heart attack, and there is no evidence that either drug reduces overall mortality in women.

Fourth, when researchers weigh the possible risks of HRT against the health benefits for women in menopause and the years after, the benefits come out way ahead. As Hodis and Mack summarized, the cardiovascular risks associated with menopausal HRT, such as stroke and thromboembolism, are rare (fewer than 10 cases in every 10,000 women) and are not unique to HRT. They are rarer and more benign than risks that occur in other commonly used medications, such as statins, aspirin, and calcium channel blockers. (We will consider the modest risks of HRT in chapter 8.)

Long before the WHI study, two analyses that weighed HRT's risks against its benefits yielded astonishing conclusions. In one calculation, 50-year-old women were assumed to take oestrogen for 25 years, to age 75. In a cohort of 10,000 women, those using oestrogen would gain nearly four additional quality-adjusted years of life compared with women not using it (because they would be much less likely to die of heart disease, hip fracture, and diabetes).[48] Another calculation concluded that HRT should increase life expectancy for nearly all postmenopausal women by three years or more, varying according to a woman's individual history and risk factors.[49]

Sometimes a retrospective investigation unexpectedly hits pay dirt. Researchers at Cedars-Sinai Medical Center in Los Angeles analyzed the coronary calcium scans (an indirect measure of plaque buildup in the arteries) of more than 4,000 women taken between 1998 and 2012. (We pause to note the influence of the Women's Health Initiative—more than 60 percent of these women were taking hormones in 1998 and only 23 percent in 2012.) After accounting for the women's ages, calcium scores, and cardiovascular risk factors, they found that women who had been taking HRT were less likely to die than those not on hormone therapy; less likely to have a coronary calcium score above 399 (indicative of severe atherosclerosis and high heart attack risk); and more likely to have the lowest possible coronary calcium score—zero—(indicating a low likelihood of heart attack).[50]

Three to four more years of healthy life with a much lower risk of heart disease? That's good enough evidence for us.

5

Breaking Bad

Avrum's mother-in-law, Charlotte, was standing alone on the granite entry outside Av's office building. Without warning, her left hip gave way and she fell to the ground. She did not lose consciousness nor feel much pain, but she was unable to get up. Charlotte was 78 years old at the time and was found to have a fracture in the neck of her femur. She had no prior history of a hip injury; it seemed that her femur had simply tired of supporting her weight. She was a healthy woman and no one, including Av, had predicted a vulnerability to fracture. On the contrary, she had dutifully taken vitamins and calcium for years and had been a champion handball player in her early life.

Osteoporosis, which means "porous bone," describes the cavities that develop in aging bones as they slowly degenerate. Bones that have been thinned out by these cavities are less able to support a person's weight, and if the bones become too thin and brittle, they can easily fracture—indeed, sometimes the simple act of bending over or even coughing will do it. Increasing bone fragility is a normal part of aging, just like cataracts, gray hair, and taking longer to recall the name of that guy you'll never forget. But osteoporosis is a different magnitude of bone loss—it's like the difference between the normal slowdown in retrieving that name and dementia.

The development of osteoporosis in later years affects men and women of all ethnicities, but the risks are higher among white and Asian women, women who are very thin, and women who enter menopause early. Women over the age of 50 have four times the rate of osteoporosis than men do, and their fractures occur five to ten years earlier than men's.[1] As people are living longer, hip fractures that result from osteoporosis are becoming more frequent; 2023 estimates are 10 million cases per year worldwide, and more than 70 percent of them occur in women.[2] Of course, osteoporosis is not the only cause of hip fractures. A woman's risk doubles if her mother had a hip fracture before age 80; other factors, such as poor eyesight and balance problems, increase the risk of falls in older people, which in turn increases the risk of fractures.[3]

Bones are living things. Like our hearts and muscles, they are not the same as they were last week or last year. Bones are in a constant state of equilibrium between the cells that build them up and those that break them down. Over a person's lifetime, that balance between growth and loss changes. Until the age of 25, more bone is formed than lost. From 25 to 30, women reach their peak bone mass, and that remains steady for the next decade. After women turn 40, bone formation slowly declines, and after they turn 50, bone loss is greater than bone formation; osteoporosis is the cumulative result.

The areas in the skeletal system where thinning bones cause the most trouble are the spinal column and the hips. The spinal column is made up of 24 individual vertebrae extending from the neck to the low back and nine fused vertebrae in the sacrum and coccyx. Each individual vertebra is separated from its neighbor above and below by a spongy disk that helps absorb the thumps and assaults of everyday life and cushions the vertebral bone. Over the course of many years, however, the vertebrae develop tiny microfractures as a result of repeated small injuries and the usual stresses of life and are slowly compressed, thereby making us shorter as we get older. When the front-facing sides of the vertebrae at the neck or upper spine wear down faster than the back sides, the vertebrae tilt forward, creating the ill-named dowager's hump at the base of the neck and upper back—a sign of advanced osteoporosis. Exercises can correct bad posture (frequently caused by the forward slumping that so many people develop from hours at the computer), but they cannot fix the anatomy of degenerated bone.

A far more serious problem than fractures of the vertebrae are hip fractures that result from a gradual weakening of the largest bones in the body, the femurs, especially the necks of the femurs, which have the daunting task of supporting the weight of the upper half of the body. Hip fractures can cause immense pain and lasting disability. Many of us can tell sorrowful stories of a healthy beloved older relative who was doing fine until she had an unexpected fall, broke her hip or pelvis, and subsequently sank into mental and physical decline.

Even more worrying, hip fractures increase the risk of death among older people. The most common estimates are that about 20 to 25 percent of the patients who have hip fractures, especially if they are in their seventies or eighties, will die within a year, and many more will suffer serious impairments in functioning.[4] In a major study headed by Danish endocrinologists, nearly 170,000 patients with hip fractures—virtually every patient in Denmark who broke a hip between 1977 and 2001—were compared with a control group, matched by age and gender, and followed for as long as twenty years from the date of injury. The mortality rate was twice as high in fracture cases as in the control group, primarily during the first year but continuing for the next five years. Perhaps that higher risk of death occurs because an old person who falls and breaks a hip is suffering from other age-related diseases? No. Although the fracture patients were more likely to have other medical problems, those problems did not affect their higher risk of death; the major reason for this higher rate was complications from the fracture. After having a hip fracture, women lost an average of 3.75 years of life. Rather dramatically, the researchers calculated that if the women were 50 or younger at the time of the fractures, they would lose 27 percent of their expected remaining years; if they were over 80, they would lose 38 percent of their expected remaining years.[5]

Two large-scale international studies echoed these mortality results. In France, researchers followed 7,512 postmenopausal women for an average of four years. The women who had a first hip fracture during that time were four times more likely to die than were those who did not have a fracture—and, again, this increase in mortality was most pronounced during the first six months following the fracture.[6] In Sweden, researchers followed 1,013 hip-fracture patients and 2,026 matched controls for, incredibly, 22 years. Twenty-one percent of the female patients died within a year of the hip fracture compared to 6 percent of the controls, and the risk of death was more than doubled for at least ten years following the hip fracture. It remained at least 50 percent higher for the duration of the 22-year observation period.[7]

Understandably, then, the prevalence of hip fractures and their consequences for impaired functioning and well-being are a major public health concern. Although rates of hip fractures have declined slightly since 1995 (for unknown reasons), the absolute numbers have increased along with the aging population. Women fear dying of breast cancer, but that risk and the lifetime risk of dying of complications of a hip fracture—primarily circulatory diseases and dementia—are about the same.[8]

Bone Density Versus Bone Resilience: A Crucial Distinction

The structure of bone is similar to the structure of a tall building. The girders that support the building are comparable to the collagen fibers within bone that provide, in addition to structural support, elasticity or tensile strength, allowing the bone to undergo stress, to bend without breaking. This flexible internal framework of the bone is called the osteoid. Calcium is deposited in and on the osteoid, creating the outer shell of the bone, like the external face of the building. The calcium in that outer shell provides a strong shield for the softer osteoid and aids the load-bearing potential of the bone, but it does not aid the bone's ability to bend without breaking.[9] An increase in calcium and other minerals, therefore, increases the stiffness and supportive strength of the bone but decreases its flexibility. As a woman ages, the thick, elastic collagen fibers inside the bone become thinner and more brittle. The tensile strength of the bone, which is a measurement of the force required to bend the bone to the point where it snaps, is diminished, and bone fractures occur more easily.

The first physician to advocate oestrogen to prevent osteoporosis was Fuller Albright, in 1940.[10] Albright was an honored endocrinologist who specialized in bone metabolism; to this day, the American Society for Bone and Mineral Research gives the Fuller Albright Award in recognition of outstanding accomplishment in the field. In 1946, Albright carefully distinguished *osteoporosis,* a disease caused by a lack of resilience within the matrix of the bone, from *osteomalacia* (known as rickets in children), caused by the bones' deficiency of minerals. With osteomalacia, the bones lack the strength conferred by calcium during a person's first two decades of life and bend on exposure to stress. (The bowlegged stance of children who grow up in impoverished areas and lack both vitamin D and calcium is characteristic of this condition.) Albright found that of his 42 patients under age 65 who had osteoporosis in the spine and the hip, 40 were postmenopausal women and only two were men. Accordingly, he named the condition *postmenopausal osteoporosis* to distinguish it from what he considered normal bone loss due to aging. But over the decades, as women began living many years past menopause and into their eighties and nineties, the condition he observed in his under-65-year-old women began to afflict many millions more.

Over time, however, some physicians began to conflate osteoporosis and osteomalacia, and the subsequent blurring of the two conditions led to the widespread but incorrect belief that if women just took enough calcium and vitamin D, they could stave off osteoporosis. It's easy to see how this mistake made its way into the culture. Even the National Library of Medicine's website advises women to take calcium and vitamins to ward off the risk of osteoporotic bone fractures.

Although calcium is crucial for the development of strong bones in children and adolescents, once bones are formed, additional calcium neither prevents nor treats bone loss. Albright had cautioned that because postmenopausal osteoporosis was not caused by any process related to the metabolism of calcium or other minerals, high intakes of these minerals with or without vitamin D would have no benefit. His observation was correct then, and it still is. Orthopedic surgeons in China performed a meta-analysis of 33 randomized trials involving 51,145 people. They evaluated the incidence of fractures in people taking supplements compared to those taking a placebo or getting no treatment. Taking calcium on its own, vitamin D on its own, or calcium plus vitamin D were not associated with a lower risk of fractures. The WHI confirmed these results in 2013 and again in 2024.[11]

The reason that calcium supplements do not reduce the risk of hip fractures is that they do not affect the interior architecture of the bone.[12] Calcium supplements affect *density* but not *resilience*—the ability of bones to bend without breaking—and it's resilience that matters here. That is why the WHI found that calcium and vitamin D supplements resulted in a small improvement in hip-bone density. But because density does not equate with resilience, the supplements did not significantly reduce the incidence of hip fracture.[13] As for the ever-popular vitamin D, save your money. A 2022 study of supplemental vitamin D given to 13,085 women ages 55 and older reported no reduced risk of fractures compared to placebo.[14] How did it become so popular? Why do media stories and many physicians continue to advise women to take it for "osteopenia" and bone health in general? The *New York Times* offered a reason in its 2018 exposé "Vitamin D, the Sunshine Supplement, Has Shadowy Money Behind It."[15]

Both oestrogen and progesterone stimulate bone formation and inhibit bone loss, and no therapy studied has proven to be better than oestrogen in preventing osteoporosis and fractures in the spine and hips. From the 1970s through the 1990s, oestrogen was the cornerstone of the prevention and treatment of osteoporosis, whether on its own or in combination with progesterone.[16] A consensus-development conference is a meeting of experts convened to assess the best medical approach to a particular problem, and two such conferences, one held at the NIH and one sponsored by the European Foundation for Osteoporosis and Bone Disease, reported that oestrogen slowed or even stopped bone loss and was the *only* well-established treatment that reduced the frequency of osteoporotic fractures in postmenopausal women.[17] Studies at the Fred Hutchinson Cancer Research Center and the Framingham study found that postmenopausal women taking oestrogen had a 35 to 50 percent reduction in the likelihood of having a fracture.[18] In the 1990s, three major studies in Sweden of many thousands of women likewise found that among those who were taking oestrogen or HRT, the risk of having a first hip fracture was significantly reduced.[19] The WHI investigators themselves acknowledged this benefit of oestrogen, reporting a 33 percent reduction in hip fractures among women on hormone therapy.[20]

Serge Rozenberg, head of the menopause and osteoporosis unit at the University Hospital of the Free University of Brussels, and his colleagues have confirmed that HRT reduces the risk of osteoporosis and of fractures. It is especially beneficial for women who reach menopause early, in their forties, because HRT also reduces the risk of cardiovascular disease, which increases in the absence of treatment.[21] (Women may enter menopause before age 50 because of surgery, chemotherapy, radiotherapy, a genetic abnormality, or for unknown reasons.)

However, for oestrogen to reduce the risk of fractures that occur ten to thirty years after menopause, postmenopausal women must be on HRT for at least ten years — and possibly for the rest of their lives. In a large clinical review of the evidence, Nananda Col and her colleagues noted that because 86 percent of hip fractures occur among women over the age of 65, women who take hormones only in their fifties, typically to alleviate menopausal symptoms, would not derive much benefit in terms of protecting their bones decades later. A few years of taking hormones, they said, would have little effect on fracture risk by the time a woman approaches the age at which that risk peaks.[22] They were right; the protective effect of hormone therapy on the bones vanishes when it is stopped, and bone loss resumes at an accelerated rate.[23] When women go off oestrogen, the risk of hip fractures rapidly increases, and within six years it is where it would have been had they never taken hormones at all.

In a review of eleven studies of oestrogen and hip fracture conducted since 1990, epidemiologist Deborah Grady and her colleagues found that all but one reported a reduction in the risk of hip fractures among women taking oestrogen compared with nonusers. Again, the longer the women had been taking oestrogen — ten years or more — the lower their risk of hip fractures.[24] And, again, that beneficial effect, even among women who had been taking oestrogen for a decade, declined rapidly after they stopped. Women ages 65 to 74 who had taken oestrogen in the past had a 63 percent reduction in the risk of hip fracture, but if they stopped taking hormones, by the time they were 75, they had only an 18 percent reduction in risk. A year after this study came out, Grady and her colleague Bruce Ettinger, an osteoporosis specialist and endocrinologist, concluded: "To provide maximal protection, oestrogen treatment may have to be started at the time of the menopause and never stopped."[25]

The primary reason that hormones were unseated as the method of choice for preventing or delaying osteoporosis was, no surprise, the WHI-inspired fear that HRT caused breast cancer. Even today, the Mayo Clinic's website states that "the reduction of oestrogen levels in women around the time of menopause is one of the strongest risk factors for developing osteoporosis....Oestrogen, especially when started soon after menopause, can help maintain bone density." Then, regrettably, it adds: "However, oestrogen therapy can increase the risk of breast cancer and blood clots, which can cause strokes."[26] As we have seen, that caution is largely unwarranted. Nevertheless, aren't there alternatives to hormones that prevent severe bone loss in old age and reduce the likelihood of hip fractures and their attendant risks?

WHAT ARE THE ALTERNATIVES?

Many health activists and historians of medicine believe that osteoporosis is not as serious a concern as it has been made out to be. After all, the vast majority of women, even in their eighties, will not suffer hip fractures, although they likely will have age-related microfractures in the spine. But losing a few inches in height hardly warrants a woman taking hormones her whole postmenopausal life, they argue. In *Aging Bones: A Short History of Osteoporosis,* medical historian Gerald N. Grob told the story of how, in his view, the "normal aging of bones was transformed into a medical diagnosis that eventually included every aged person."[27] This transformation, he maintained, occurred "through a coalition of cultural, medical and pharmaceutical forces that moved osteoporosis from the margins of health research in the earlier part of the twentieth century to the centre of a national and well-funded American agenda by the twenty-first century." The result was that all women over 65 and all men over 70 were urged to get bone mineral density screens. Grob showed that during the 1950s and 1960s, as more and more people were living to the age of 65 and beyond, they found themselves facing new health concerns created by additional years of life. At the same time, they were emerging as an identifiable group with distinct views, one of which was a vehement rejection of old age as a gloomy time of infirmity and disability. Accordingly, wrote Grob, "preventing age-related decline became a focus for researchers and clinicians alike."

Grob had no quarrel with helping old people live healthier lives; his concern was society's labeling the normal changes that occur with age, including menopause and bone loss, as diagnosable "diseases." Osteoporosis and its treatment, Grob argued, were "shaped by illusions about the conquest of disease and aging. These illusions, in turn, are instrumental in shaping our health care system. While bone density tests and osteoporosis treatments are now routinely prescribed, aggressive pharmaceutical intervention has produced results that are inconclusive at best."

We agree with Grob in his assessment of the cultural manufacture of new diseases that allegedly warrant drugs that Big Pharma just coincidentally happens to have developed. We too lament the American pursuit of youth and the illusions of conquering age. But the search for treatments to help the millions who are at risk of suffering or premature death, precisely because they are living longer than would once have been dreamed possible, is another matter entirely. Alzheimer's disease and other forms of dementia also afflict people living into old age; should we not do all we can to understand the causes of these disorders and thereby prevent or treat them?

For their part, many women are uncomfortable with the idea of taking any medication for their entire lives after menopause. Even Ettinger and Grady, who found that the improvement in bone resilience conferred by oestrogen was likely to reduce the risk of fracture by about two-thirds, worried that "having to take oestrogen for the rest of one's life reduces the appeal of this preventive strategy." Some writers suggest that only women at very high risk of bone fractures should consider HRT. Everyone else should look first to alternatives: Exercise. Take fluoride. Take calcium. Take medication designed to prevent osteoporosis, namely bisphosphonates. If only it were that easy.

Exercise, the most popular recommended alternative to hormones for bone strength, is a fine activity for many health reasons; weight training in particular is of undeniable benefit to women as they age. Some investigators have suggested that peak bone strength can be achieved by a combination of exercise and calcium during a woman's premenopausal years, while she has adequate levels of circulating oestrogen, and that an elevated peak bone strength might stave off or delay future osteoporosis. Exercises that maintain muscle strength, endurance, and balance can indeed lower the risk of falling—the leading cause of hip fracture. But they do not reliably improve bone flexibility in postmenopausal women who are not on HRT.[28]

Because fluoride protects the outer shell of our teeth, some investigators have tried it as a treatment for women with osteoporosis, administering it in large doses to prevent further deterioration of bones. Fluoride does generate dramatic increases in bone density but it does not improve bone tensile strength, probably because it makes the bones less flexible.[29]

Well, then, what alternatives might increase bone flexibility? Bone density can be measured, but the more relevant bone fragility—the bones' response to tensile stress—cannot. The best way to test the tensile strength of bone would be to clamp the bone in a vise and determine how much bending the bone could tolerate before it breaks. Clearly, this is not a practical method! Physicians therefore use a bone mineral density (BMD) test as a substitute for measuring the tensile strength of bone, but they often overlook the fact that this test is an inaccurate measure of fracture risk.[30] (The BMD's accuracy may be enhanced by adding a Trabecular Bone Score, an indirect indicator of bone microarchitecture.) Today the most commonly used test is dual-energy X-ray absorptiometry (DXA), which uses X-rays to measure the amounts of calcium and other minerals in the bone. But it too is measuring bone density, not bone resilience.

BMD tests were supported by the pharmaceutical industry, and Gerry Grob, along with other bioethicists, medical historians, and consumer advocates, warned that once the tests were in widespread use, they would open the door for new medications for osteoporosis.

Before a company can sell a drug, after all, it must have a condition or disease that the medication treats. Therefore, it must have a way of identifying that disease. And if a company can cast a wide net in its definition of that disease, it'll have an even larger market of people to take its new drug, as we saw with new definitions of high cholesterol and statins. But where along the continuum of bone loss—which, after all, happens to everyone—does it become a disease? How little is too much?

The ensuing commercial campaign to simplify the decision to prescribe medication began with an arbitrary answer: on the continuum of bone loss, a person whose bone mineral density test score is 2.5 standard deviations below that of a healthy 30-year-old will meet the (artificial) diagnosis of osteoporosis. (A standard deviation is a statistical measure that describes the distance, or deviation, from the norm.) In the early 1990s, this numerical criterion was endorsed by the World Health Organization, and with that official imprimatur, researchers and clinicians had a tangible number to hold on to.[31] That -2.5 diagnostic threshold, wrote Bruce Ettinger and his colleagues, was simply a benchmark for estimating the prevalence of osteoporosis across various countries. "It was not intended," they wrote, "to be the sole clinical criterion for determining drug treatment. Intervention thresholds differ from diagnostic thresholds."[32]

But wait—if -2.5 is bad, isn't -2.0 or -1.5 pre-bad? What if your score is less than that normal 30-year-old's but not officially osteoporotic? That can't be good for you, can it? A new diagnosis to the rescue: the term *osteopenia* emerged, defined as a BMD test result between -1.0 and -2.5 standard deviations below that of a healthy 30-year-old. Osteopenia was assumed to be an inevitable precursor of osteoporosis, just as a puppy is a pre-dog. The World Health Organization emphasized that this diagnostic category was not meant to be used in clinical practice, because *osteopenia* has no clinical significance and does not even predict the risk for osteoporotic fracture. Canadian physicians and health-policy specialists Angela Cheung and Allan Detsky reported that a history of falls is a stronger predictor of fractures than bone mineral density results, which do not correlate well with the risk of hip fracture.[33] The term *osteopenia* has "no medical meaning," Steven Cummings, an epidemiologist who has conducted numerous large-scale studies, told a reporter. "I've seen patients who come in scared that they will become disabled soon because they have this 'disease' called osteopenia, when in fact they are normal for their age."[34] Nortin M. Hadler, professor emeritus of medicine and microbiology/immunology at the University of North Carolina and author of several books on medical overtreatment, was even more forthright. "Osteopenia is an example of a New Age social construction," he said, adding that it was invented and sustained by marketers, drug companies, and others with vested interests.[35]

Too late for the warnings; there was too much money at stake. Gynecologists began buying expensive DXA machines to use on their patients; Carol's doctor told her she had osteopenia but then had the grace to smile and say, "Although that doesn't mean anything." Prescriptions for bisphosphonates, seen as an alternative to HRT to ward off bone loss, skyrocketed, now being used to treat both the meaningless osteopenia and the true condition of osteoporosis. Ever since the Women's Health Initiative, the preventive treatment of osteoporosis has been dominated by nonhormonal bisphosphonates such as Fosamax, Aredia, Actonel, Zometa, Reclast, and Boniva.[36] These come in oral and intravenous forms and can be taken daily, weekly, monthly, or even annually. Bisphosphonates do nothing for the nonexistent condition of osteopenia, but they can avert osteoporosis in women at high risk and also stabilize bone loss in women who already have it. Once osteoporosis has developed, however, it is highly unlikely that the drugs can reverse the condition.

The side effects of the bisphosphonates can be unpleasant, and some are far worse than those for hormones. The most common are abdominal discomfort, muscle or joint pain, fever and flulike symptoms, and insomnia; two very rare but devastating side effects are kidney damage and osteonecrosis of the jaw, a disease presumed to be caused by a diminished flow of blood to the bone in that area. No wonder that among patients with osteoporosis, including those who have had fractures, 70 percent stop the medication within a year.[37]

Worse, when the bisphosphonates are taken for long periods, they have been associated with an *increased* risk of atypical hip fractures. Unlike hip fractures caused by osteoporosis, which usually occur at the angled upper extension (the neck) of the femur, atypical femoral fractures generally develop below the femoral neck in the upper part of the shaft. Taking bisphosphonates over the long term may impair the bones' ability to repair microcracks, thereby leading to increased skeletal fragility.[38] In 2017, the Women's Health Initiative announced that in older women at high risk of fracture, taking bisphosphonates for ten to thirteen years was associated with a higher risk of clinical fracture than two years of use.[39]

All of this evidence led epidemiologist Robert Langer, the WHI critic, to argue that oestrogen was a better preventive: "Unlike bisphosphonates, which have been associated with excessive bone mineralization, oestrogen facilitates normal bone architecture. There is no question that oestrogen is an effective and metabolically appropriate preventive strategy for osteoporotic fractures, and that osteoporosis is a chronic disease with tremendous impact in postmenopausal women."[40]

The pharmaceutical industry is not sitting around quietly resting on its bisphosphonates, you can be sure. Many drug companies have entered the race for other ways to prevent or treat osteoporosis. Consider these alternatives to bisphosphonates:

Raloxifene (Evista), a SERM (selective (o)estrogen-receptor modulator), is prescribed for some postmenopausal, oestrogen-receptor-positive breast cancer survivors to decrease the risk of breast cancer recurrence. Raloxifene, which has been used for many years to treat osteoporosis, decreases the risk of vertebral fractures but it does not reduce the risk of hip fractures.[41] About a fourth of the women who take it report hot flushes, and 10 to 20 percent report flulike symptoms, sinusitis, joint pains, and muscle spasms.

Calcitonin, a hormone produced in the thyroid gland, helps regulate the blood's calcium and phosphate levels. It is generally administered by nasal spray or injection. It may help reduce bone loss, but there is no substantive evidence that it reduces the risk of fractures.[42]

Teriparatide (Forteo), a form of parathyroid hormone generated from recombinant DNA, stimulates bone growth and reduces the risk of hip fractures in patients who have already developed osteoporosis.[43] However, its protective effects wane after two years of continued treatment. Abaloparatide, a chemical cousin of Forteo, does reduce the risk of vertebral fractures, but its effectiveness for hip fractures is still unclear.[44]

Denosumab (Prolia or Xgeva), approved for the treatment of osteoporosis and to decrease fractures caused by metastases of cancer to the bone, has a similar rate of success as the bisphosphonates in reducing the risk of vertebral and hip fractures. It must be taken indefinitely, and few patients are willing to do that. Nearly half of the women who take this drug report side effects of fatigue and weakness; about 20 percent report shortness of breath, coughing, and muscle and joint pain. A dangerous drop in calcium levels has been reported in a small percentage of cancer patients treated with denosumab.[45]

Of all these efforts to develop the best drug, the story of romosozumab is perhaps the most instructive. Romosozumab, developed by Celltech and marketed by Amgen, binds to and inhibits sclerostin, a protein that leads to bone resorption (loss). There was great excitement in 2017 when a study of the drug that included nearly 4,100 postmenopausal women with osteoporosis appeared in the *New England Journal of Medicine*. The accompanying editorial was titled "Romosozumab — Promising or Practice Changing?" The women were randomly assigned to receive the newer drug or Fosamax for twelve months, followed by another year of Fosamax for everyone. The researchers then looked to see how many women had developed new fractures at twenty-four months. The results sure seemed "practice changing." After two years, the romosozumab-to-Fosamax group had nearly half the risk of developing new vertebral fractures (6.2 percent) than the Fosamax-only group (11.9 percent), and a lower risk of hip fractures as well.[46]

The research was funded by Amgen. In that same year, the FDA rejected the drugmaker's application for approval because the drug also caused an increased risk of "serious adverse cardiovascular events." As one article reported: "Safety concerns could limit the label of romosozumab and in doing so dent its blockbuster ambitions. 'Ultimately based on a label that fits the right risk/benefit population and based on conversations with Amgen, we still think the drug could be a $500M+ franchise,' Jefferies analyst Michael Yee wrote in a note to investors."[47]

Did you get that "blockbuster ambitions" part? The drug company has since regrouped and won FDA approval for the drug for postmenopausal women with osteoporosis who are at risk of bone fracture. A 2022 review paper noted that "the lack of long-term trials and data warrants continued monitoring of patients taking romosozumab" to evaluate for "potential adverse effects."[48] Meaning: *We got the drug approved fast, and we'll see if there are risks we didn't notice with short-term testing.* A few other problems with the drug remain — its high cost, the necessity for monthly appointments to receive the injection, and osteonecrosis of the jaw. And, oh, yes, after a year, its effects wane and bone mineral density returns to baseline.

The Take-Home

We are mindful of the irony that while we are busy criticizing Big Pharma for hurrying new drugs to market, exaggerating their benefits, and minimizing their risks, we are advocating the use of hormone therapies that are manufactured by Big Pharma companies. We are not happy that Wyeth, which has held the patent on

Premarin for sixty years, has fought in court to prevent generic formulations from being marketed. Because Wyeth controls this drug, which is the most widely prescribed oestrogen, it has been able to increase its price. We deplore this action, by Wyeth or any other drug company. But reprehensible marketing practices do not necessarily negate a drug's benefits, and Premarin's safety and efficacy record stretches back for decades.

As an oncologist and hematologist who has been in medical practice for fifty years, Avrum knows full well that no physician can read and evaluate every article that appears in the medical literature and that some research will be inconsistent with the conclusions that he or she comes to. In the case of HRT's benefits for bone health, his conclusions are the result of decades of assessing research findings, his accumulated clinical experience, his debates with respected colleagues, and the constant input from his peers and his patients. Given present knowledge, he feels that these conclusions are warranted:

- Osteoporosis and subsequent bone fracture with resulting disability and death are growing problems for the expanding population of women living into their seventies, eighties, and nineties.
- Currently, oestrogen is the most effective intervention with the fewest unpleasant or dire side effects for preventing or diminishing the development of osteoporosis. It has been repeatedly shown to reduce the risk of the condition's most incapacitating complication, hip fracture, by 30 to 50 percent. In absolute numbers, this reduction is highly meaningful.

- Exercise may improve bone strength and resistance to fracture in premenopausal women, but it does not improve bone strength or resistance to fracture among postmenopausal women who are not on HRT.
- Calcium supplements and vitamin D, which millions of women take in hopes of fending off loss of bone density, are ineffective in preventing postmenopausal osteoporosis or fractures because they do not affect bone *resilience*.
- The most frequently prescribed nonhormonal osteoporosis medications, the bisphosphonates, are associated with gastrointestinal discomfort, fatigue, and insomnia; with an increased risk of atypical femoral fractures if taken for a long time; and with the rare but debilitating development of kidney problems or osteonecrosis of the jaw.

The prevention of osteoporosis may not be the leading and best reason for women to take HRT; Gerry Grob and other critics of medicalization are right, after all, that the vast majority of women will not develop this condition or die of it. But the research persuades us that women who are at high risk of osteoporosis should continue taking hormones indefinitely once they are past menopause. And for those who decide to take HRT for the many other benefits it confers, having stronger and more resilient bones certainly seems to be one hell of a welcome side effect.

6

Losing and Using Our Minds

Dear Dr. Bluming:

When the Danish study came out in July 2023, I stopped using HRT immediately. The study certainly scared me. When I stopped HRT, my symptoms returned tenfold. I would really, really like to go back to utilizing the gel, but I'm just not sure what to do. I've read about HRT benefitting cognition and brain health and had felt good about using it prior to this study. What should I do? How reliable is that study?

This writer was not alone. The "Danish study" immediately generated anxiety about a possible connection between HRT and cognitive decline. That is not remotely what the study actually found, as we will show you at the end of this chapter. But there is no question that worries about dementia are front and center for many people. We remember one particularly ominous headline in huge type on the front page of the Sunday Review section of the *New York Times* on November 19, 2017: "Is Alzheimer's Coming for You?" Followed by the slug: "Simple blood tests may soon be able to deliver alarming news about your cognitive health." Oh, goody.

The article sure grabbed our attention. It reported that anywhere from one-fourth to one-half of the population will show signs of Alzheimer's disease by age 85, a risk that is even higher among people carrying one or two copies of the gene variant APOE4 (apolipoprotein E4). The article raised the possibility of a future blood test that would be easier and less expensive than gene sequencing, a test that could identify pre-Alzheimer's in 40- to 50-year-old people who have no obvious symptoms. Pagan Kennedy, the reporter, interviewed research scientists who were studying Alzheimer's causes as well as people who knew they had the gene variant and had joined support groups, seeking diet and lifestyle interventions in hopes of preventing or at least slowing the progression of the disease. One neurologist, David Holtzman, had been studying the APOE gene for twenty-five years without looking to see if he had the APOE4 variant. When Kennedy asked him why he hadn't, he told her there was no point because there was no drug or lifestyle program guaranteed to protect the brain.

Alzheimer's disease is one of many conditions that fall under the umbrella term *dementia*. Right behind women's fear of breast cancer is the fear of "losing it": losing memory, clear thinking, words. (A fear that men share, of course.) Everyone becomes forgetful: "Where are those keys? Why did I come into the den—was I looking for something?" Cognitive slowdown is normal as we age;

we *will* remember the name of that actor who played in that film we liked so much...wait, what was it called?...but it will take us longer than we'd like. Mild cognitive slowdown is variously exasperating and amusing, but for people entering their sixties and seventies, the prospect of dementia is terrifying: "If I can't remember now where I put my car keys, does that mean that one day I won't remember what car keys are for?" Many people fear so, but these are very different matters. A sign of dementia is memory loss that disrupts daily life: forgetting recently learned information and important dates, asking for the same information over and over, relying on family members for reminders of events the person could once easily handle. But merely forgetting names or appointments for a while and remembering them eventually are typical changes that occur with age.

In 1900, only 5 percent of all American women lived beyond their fiftieth birthday; today their average life expectancy has reached 80. For women now age 45, the estimated lifetime risk for developing Alzheimer's dementia is one in five; it's one in ten for men. One reason for women's higher risk is their longer life span, since rates of Alzheimer's dementia increase dramatically with age; but even after controlling for their greater longevity, women are still more likely than men to develop the disease. Almost two-thirds of all people with Alzheimer's are women, and a woman in her sixties is twice as likely to develop Alzheimer's as she is to develop breast cancer. Because the overall population continues to age, with more and more people living well past their eighties, the number of people who die from Alzheimer's disease every year has almost doubled even while deaths from other diseases—notably breast cancer, prostate cancer, stroke, and heart disease—are in decline. Someone in the United States develops Alzheimer's disease every 66 seconds, and by 2050, barring scientific discoveries, it will be one new case every 33 seconds — 13 million people.[1]

Because Alzheimer's patients typically survive from four to eight years after the onset of the illness (with some living as long as twenty years more, reflecting, as the Alzheimer's Association says, its "slow, insidious, and uncertain" course), the cost of their care to families and society is immense, financially as well as emotionally. With about six and a half million Americans currently living with Alzheimer's, the total cost for their health care, including long-term care and hospice services, reached $345 billion in 2023. (For comparison, that is about $130 billion more than the cost of care for people with all cancers combined.)

Given the suffering that Alzheimer's causes, the misery it inflicts on families, and the financial burden it imposes, it's no wonder that attempts to prevent it, control it, and treat it are a high priority. Scientists are investigating all kinds of possible causes, including genetics, exposure to environmental toxins and pollution, cardiovascular problems, and chronic inflammation. And yet almost nothing is known for sure. Because the only way to accurately diagnose it is by microscopic assessment of the brain after death, the diagnosis in living persons is not definitive. Alzheimer's might prove to be a family of illnesses rather than one.

To date, no drug has succeeded in preventing or slowing the development of dementia. Yet there is evidence that one preventive, at least for women, is right under our noses: oestrogen. Decades of research have demonstrated its role in helping to preserve the cognitive ability of postmenopausal women and in decreasing the risk of Alzheimer's.[2] But, as usual, the WHI weighed in with a contrary view. In 2003, the WHI Memory Study (WHIMS) reported that oestrogen plus progestin nearly doubled the relative risk for dementia in women 65 and older—further support, the investigators said, for their warning that the risks of HRT outweighed any possible benefits.[3] There they go again. Doubled the risk? Well, the investigators admitted, "the absolute risk is relatively small." The risk increased from 1 percent (21 out of 2,303) of the women on placebo to 1.8 percent (40 out of 2,229) of the women on HRT.

That was enough. In one fell swoop, all of the accumulated knowledge disputing that conclusion was rejected in favor of a small statistical finding of questionable significance, and millions of women were denied the potential benefit of HRT in warding off the cognitive decline that so often accompanies aging.

Still, nearly double is nearly double, so let's look closely at the basis of the WHI's claim. At the outset, the researchers had an admirable goal: They would select 8,300 women, all over age 65, from the original, much larger WHI sample to be part of their memory study. (Thus, these women were not representative of the vast majority of women in the general population; most women who decide to take hormones usually start them when they enter menopause.) They would follow these women for five years to see who developed cognitive impairments and whether hormones increased their risk. The large size of the group—more than 8,000—would allow them to draw statistically reliable conclusions.

However, this ambition was thwarted, because when the WHI ended the HRT part of the trial early, with those stop-the-presses claims of an increased risk of breast cancer, they had just 4,532 women enrolled. Of that number, only 61 had developed dementia over four years. Undeterred by the few cases that might throw their calculations into question, the researchers justified the low number as being "in keeping with both the age of the cohort and the expectation that healthier, cognitively and behaviorally competent women were more likely to have enrolled in this complex and rigorously conducted clinical trial."[4] This is hardly a satisfying explanation for many reasons, starting with the fact that the great majority of the women in their sample were *not* healthier. (You may recall that 70 percent were overweight or obese, half were smokers, and many had hypertension.) Whatever the reason for the low number of women who developed dementia during the study, it means that any difference between the HRT group and the placebo group—that 1 percent versus 1.8 percent—could be statistically significant while at the same time being neither compelling nor clinically relevant.

The investigators claimed to have identified an elephant that on closer inspection turned out to be a mouse. Here is one of our favorite lines: "In the WHIMS," the authors began, and then they paused midsentence to interject a self-congratulatory pat on the back—"the first double-blind, placebo-controlled, long-term multicenter study of [oestrogen alone and HRT] in postmenopausal women"—*both* forms of hormone therapy "were associated with an increased incidence of dementia compared with placebo." That sounds bad, but the sentence continued: "although the association did not reach statistical significance in the smaller, but longer, oestrogen-alone trial."[5] Talking out of both sides of their mouths in a single sentence, they told us there was an "increased incidence," but never mind, it was not significant for the oestrogen users. What about women taking combined oestrogen and progestin? Now they trumpeted that nearly doubled relative risk while admitting that the absolute risk was very low. But then they said the increased risk appeared during the first year that women were taking HRT, suggesting that many of these participants already had cognitive decline at the start of the study. That means the investigators were fully aware that their tested population was perhaps not quite as healthy as they had boasted.

Trying to sort out the WHI's conclusions about oestrogen and cognitive function is like playing whack-a-mole: bop one of their overblown risks on the head, and another pops up somewhere else. Sometimes the investigators talked about "dementia," sometimes "mild cognitive impairment," and sometimes, grandly, "global cognitive function." Sometimes they twisted their data into contortions to eke out a finding. In 2004, when the investigators reported that women taking oestrogen alone did not have an increased risk of dementia, they combined them with women taking oestrogen and progestin — that is, they pooled the data from both groups — and in this way, they could report a slight increased risk of dementia for both.[6] How can that be so if the women on oestrogen alone didn't have a greater risk?

As for that slightly increased risk of dementia for women on HRT: Most damning for the WHI's assertion, in that first 2003 report, there was no increased incidence of mild cognitive impairment between the HRT and placebo groups. This presented a problem: Given that "mild cognitive impairment" precedes the emergence of full-blown dementia, how could HRT cause the more serious disease but not its less serious precursor? You may recall the WHI tried the same trick with their illogical claim that HRT increases the risk of lung cancer deaths but not of actual lung cancer. Likewise, if HRT were really harmful to the brain, surely mild cognitive problems would emerge first—the warning warble of the canary in a mental mine.

The following year, 2004, the investigators must have heard that warble. This time they decided to look at the women's "global cognitive function." Both oestrogen alone and HRT, they reported, were indeed associated with cognitive impairments, *but only among women who were already cognitively impaired at the outset.* When women who had mild cognitive impairment at the start of the study were excluded from analysis, the results were no longer statistically significant. "No other factors appear to markedly influence the treatment effects of [HRT] or pooled hormone therapy," they wrote. "Among women whose scores exceeded 95 [normal cognitive ability], the mean decrement was small and not statistically different from zero."[7]

Translation: The cognitively healthy women on HRT did not become cognitively impaired!

Within a year, many of the WHI's critics had mobilized. Obstetrician-gynecologist Leon Speroff, whose anger at the WHI's statistical shenanigans we previously described, noted that "in the canceled oestrogen-progestin arm of the WHI, the only increase in dementia was in the group of women who were 75 years and older when they started treatment."[8] Somehow that finding got lost in the WHI's press releases about women's dementia risks on HRT. Neuroscientists James Simpkins and Meharvan Singh, along with a team of neurobiologists, endocrinologists, and clinical scientists who specialized in oestrogen research (including Roberta Brinton, Pauline Maki, and Barbara Sherwin), wrote a position paper critical of the WHI's claims. They observed that the results flew in the face of hundreds of studies conducted over a decade, many cited by the WHI investigators themselves, suggesting that oestrogen could protect brain cells from damage and improve cognition in people and animals. The finding of the WHI memory study, they said, had been greatly exaggerated; the small increase in dementia risk could not be extended to all forms of HRT or even to the younger women most likely to start HRT.[9]

Once again, it seems that the WHI investigators were doing their best to interpret their elusive findings in the most negative way, and they were doing so by manipulating the numbers, redefining the outcomes (mild impairment to dementia to "global cognitive function"), and claiming that HRT caused cognitive impairments for all women rather than, specifically, for the very old and those who already had cognitive deficits. This was especially curious because they began their first paper with a litany of studies demonstrating oestrogen's protective effects on the brain, including its ability to reduce the loss of neurons, improve cerebral blood flow, and modulate expression of the APOE gene.[10] Eventually, the WHI investigators conceded that their study was not designed to determine whether women who began taking oestrogen at the time of menopause would have a lower risk of the onset of cognitive decline or Alzheimer's disease a decade or two later.[11] The WHI proposed that "there may be a critical period during which hormone therapy must be initiated to protect cognitive functioning."[12] As we will see, there most certainly is.

Unfortunately, the worry that HRT increases the risk of dementia has survived among numerous physicians, even those who now recognize the limitations of many of the WHI's other scare findings. "My doctor won't prescribe HRT for me," one of Av's former patients, whom we will call Sarah, wrote to him. "He now agrees that it doesn't cause breast cancer, but he told me that the WHI says it increases the risk of dementia, and he wants to protect me from that." Protect her? Didn't this physician speak to her? If he had, he might have learned that Sarah had been on hormones for many years and that she was, at age 78, still running her own demanding business.

Was oestrogen a contributor to Sarah's healthy mental functioning, or does Sarah just have good genes, good workouts, and good habits? Scientists have three ways of investigating that question: they examine the anatomical and neurological changes in the brain that occur with impaired cognition and that oestrogen might influence; they do research on animals; and they conduct human studies that examine the effects of oestrogen on women's thinking and abilities in real life.

LESSONS FROM LABS

During the final third of the twentieth century, medical students were taught that human beings were born with a finite number of brain neurons (nerve cells), that the huge number of glial cells that surrounded them had no function other than to support the neurons in some vague way, that neurons did not divide or regenerate, and that everyone irreplaceably lost countless numbers of them every day. We now know that all of these claims are wrong. Brain neurons are capable of dividing and regenerating, and brain function depends crucially not only on neurons but also on the glial cells.* *Glia* is from the Greek word for "glue," but these cells do more than glue neurons together. They provide the neurons with nutrients, insulate them, help them grow, protect the brain from toxic agents, and remove cellular debris when neurons die. They can even evolve into neurons. Without glia, neurons could not function effectively. Over time, glia help determine which neural connections get stronger or weaker, suggesting that they play a vital role in learning and memory.

One of the most astonishing advances in brain science has been the discovery of the human brain's *neuroplasticity*, the fact that neurons can form new connections throughout a person's life, sometimes compensating for injury or disease. Laboratory studies have suggested that oestrogen can enhance neuroplasticity by modifying the structure of nerve cells in the brain and altering the way they communicate with one another. The real-life applications of this research remain uncertain, but we want to describe here some of the abundant evidence that oestrogen, administered when menopause begins, may prevent, or at least delay, the onset of dementia, including dementia resulting from Alzheimer's disease.[13] Oestrogen levels drop dramatically in women after menopause, so if oestrogen is playing a role in protecting the brain's neurons and glia, and that drop in oestrogen is one of the major contributors to women's higher rate of Alzheimer's, it behooves us to pay attention.

Researchers have identified numerous anatomical aberrations in the brains of patients with Alzheimer's disease, notably pathology

---

* Scientists used to think that the human brain contained about a hundred billion neurons and ten times as many glia. But thanks to recent advances, researchers can count individual cells, and they put the numbers much lower—an adult brain contains around 171 billion cells, about evenly divided between neurons and glia.

in specific areas involved in memory: the prefrontal cortex (active during short-term memory, and the part of the brain involved in planning and higher mental functions), the hippocampus and related areas responsible for learning and retrieving stored information, and the amygdala (involved in forming, retrieving, and consolidating emotional memories). A person can have severe abnormalities in these areas and still be able to walk, talk, and taste without remembering the name of the person sitting across the dinner table. These pathological findings include the following:

- The death of nerve cells and a decreased density of those cells.
- Thinning and atrophy of the dendrites and axons, which extend outward from the body of a nerve cell like the arms of an octopus, conveying signals that allow nerve cells to communicate with one another.
- A decreased number of synapses (the connections between neurons).
- Neurofibrillary tangles, a primary marker of Alzheimer's; these are clusters of twisted fibers inside the neurons that consist primarily of a protein called tau, which is involved in transporting nutrients from one part of the neuron to another.
- Amyloid plaques, another Alzheimer's marker (clusters of disintegrated protein fragments that build up between nerve cells).
- Decreased stores within the neuron of acetylcholine, a chemical that allows messages to leap from one neuron to the next in regions of the memory centers of the brain, especially the hippocampus, and in other regions that affect memory and

emotion. Patients with Alzheimer's disease have up to a 90 percent reduction in the level of this neurotransmitter.

• Dysfunction of the glial cells.

Researchers still disagree about whether these aberrations directly *cause* Alzheimer's or whether they are a *result* of Alzheimer's, and either way, administering oestrogen to women who already are afflicted with the disease does not help them. However, there is considerable evidence that oestrogen's effects on the brain might indeed play a significant role in preventing dementia, because oestrogen affects all of these aspects of brain anatomy, both directly and indirectly. It stimulates the growth of neurons and synapses, and it increases plasticity, the brain's remarkable ability to adapt and change.[14]

It turns out that oestrogen receptors are located throughout the brain, especially in the hippocampus and other areas involved in learning and memory.[15] Neuroscientists such as Elizabeth Gould, who is at the Princeton Neuroscience Institute, have shown that oestrogen affects the brain mechanisms involved in memory, aging, and degenerative diseases in various ways.[16] In one early study, Gould and her colleagues removed the ovaries of adult female rats, which caused levels of circulating oestrogen to plummet, which in turn decreased the number of dendrites on neurons in the rats' hippocampi. When they gave the rats oestrogen, with or without progesterone, after removing the ovaries, this decrease did not occur.[17] Similarly, when female rats are given oestrogen, the number of synapses within the hippocampus increases, they learn to run through mazes more quickly (and remember where the food is), and their neurons, especially those involved in memory, are more likely to survive during normal aging or exposure to toxins. Treating female rats with oestrogen prolongs their survival, improves their spatial-recognition memory, and decreases the amount of amyloid in neurons.[18]

Roberta Diaz Brinton, another leading neuroscientist in this field, is director of the Center for Innovation in Brain Science at the University of Arizona, where she studies the aging female brain and, in particular, how to prevent or delay Alzheimer's. In studies comparing oestrogen-treated cells to cells not exposed to oestrogen, she found significantly greater growth of dendrites and axons among the oestrogen-treated cells as well as enhanced connections among brain cells.[19]

Oestrogen has even more benefits for the brain:

- Oestrogen increases the levels of an enzyme needed to synthesize acetylcholine.[20]
- Oestrogen stimulates the growth of nerve cells, regenerates axons, and decreases the nerve-cell death that happens in Alzheimer's.[21]
- Oestrogen prevents a dangerous accumulation of calcium within the nerve cells.[22]
- Oestrogen makes brain cells more responsive and sensitive to the effects of nerve growth factor, a protein responsible for the development of new neurons and the health of mature ones.[23] (We interrupt this list to insert a remarkable story: Nerve growth factor was discovered in the 1950s by the pioneering Italian neurobiologist Rita Levi-Montalcini, a Holocaust survivor who did her original research under her bed

while hiding from the Nazis. She and colleague Stanley Cohen won the Nobel Prize for their work. Levi-Montalcini died in 2012 at the age of 103.)

- Oestrogen reduces the production of beta amyloid, the substance that accumulates in amyloid plaques.[24]
- Oestrogen prevents the buildup of the tau protein.[25]
- Oestrogen enhances the action of glial cells[26] and their ability to regulate inflammatory responses after brain injury.[27]
- Oestrogen improves cerebral blood flow. In women who have extremely low oestrogen levels because of illness or surgery, their blood-flow patterns resemble those of patients with mild to moderate Alzheimer's. In one study, administering oestrogen reversed these detrimental blood-flow changes and restored a normal pattern after only six weeks.[28]
- Oestrogen promotes the uptake of glucose and its metabolism in the brain. When women begin going through menopause and oestrogen declines, so do the glucose levels in their brains. Why does this matter? Although the brain takes up only 2 percent of a person's body weight, it uses some 20 percent of the body's glucose — the fuel of energy.[29]

Neuropsychologists Susan Resnick, Pauline Maki, and their colleagues at the National Institute of Aging used PET scans to trace blood flow in the brains of 32 women, 15 of whom were on oestrogen and 17 of whom were not, while they took tests of verbal and visual memory. (PET scans are expensive and time-consuming, so researchers have to rely on small samples to test their early hypotheses about the biological underpinnings of cognition.) The oestrogen users showed increased blood flow in the hippocampus and other brain regions involved in memory.[30] This evidence, which suggests a biological effect of oestrogen on the brain, bolsters the behavioral evidence that comes from women's performance on memory tests. As Maki said to an interviewer, "The fact that we found effects in the hippocampus makes it especially compelling."[31] The blood-flow findings suggest one route, though by no means the only one, by which oestrogen protects against memory loss.

In sum, brain and animal studies support the conclusion that memory, neurotransmitter function, brain plasticity, blood flow, glucose metabolism, and neural protection are all enhanced by oestrogen. Good news, but does it apply to women who take oestrogen for longer than a short-lived lab study?

LESSONS FROM REAL LIFE

In 1952, in one of the earliest controlled studies of the effects of oestrogen on women's cognitive functioning, Bettye McDonald Caldwell and Robert I. Watson tested 28 women, average age 75, who were living in a retirement home. They gave the women two well-established tests of verbal and other cognitive abilities—the Wechsler-Bellevue Intelligence Scale and the Wechsler Memory Scale—and then randomly assigned them to receive an injection of either oestrogen or a placebo, administered once a week for a year, at which time the women were tested again. The results were impressive: The women who were taking oestrogen during that year had a marked increase in their verbal IQ score on the intelligence and memory tests, whereas those given placebo showed a decrease on both measures of verbal ability. A year later, following withdrawal of oestrogen, the scores of all of these women had decreased back to their original baseline, indicating that oestrogen's enhancement of memory occurred only while they were taking the hormone.[32]

In 1973, in another study of 75-year-old women living in a home for the aged, Herman Kantor and his colleagues randomly assigned 25 women to be given Premarin and 25 to be given a placebo, daily, for three years. Every three months, they compared the women's scores on the Hospital Adjustment Scale, which measures behavior in three categories: communication and relationships, ability to take care of oneself, and work activities. The scores of the women on Premarin increased steadily for eighteen months and remained stable for the duration of the study; the scores of those who were given the placebo decreased steadily over time.[33] These well-controlled studies provided the first compelling evidence that oestrogen enhanced or maintained verbal abilities, verbal memory, and aspects of social and physical functioning in women's everyday lives beyond the laboratory.

In the ensuing decades, the evidence from larger studies and from other kinds of studies piled up, beginning with a groundbreaking 1988 study by psychologist Barbara Sherwin at McGill University.[34] Sherwin studied the effects of oestrogen on women's cognitive functioning for several decades, and three of her early studies were especially influential. In the first, she worked with women who had undergone surgery to remove the ovaries and uterus, so their oestrogen levels were very low. She randomly assigned some of them to be given oestrogen and the rest a placebo, and she immediately noticed a big difference. "Women who were given a placebo after their surgery complained of not being able to remember things, of having to make lists, which they never needed to do in the past. They also had lower scores on tests of verbal memory," she told a McGill reporter.[35] One test involves reading a standard paragraph and then recalling the content, a measure of short-term memory. Participants wait an hour or two, doing other things, and then try to recall the paragraph again, a measure of longer-term memory. Women who received oestrogen after surgery performed better on tests of verbal memory and other cognitive functions than women who were given the placebo.

A few years later, Sherwin and her colleague Stuart Phillips conducted a study of otherwise healthy women who had had hysterectomies and removal of their ovaries for benign disease. The women took a battery of memory tests before surgery and again two months later after receiving injections of either oestrogen or placebo. Those receiving oestrogen either stayed at their pre-surgery cognitive level or, on one test, actually improved; those on placebo did worse on most of the verbal tests.[36]

And in a third study, Sherwin and Togas Tulandi, a research scientist and chief of McGill's department of obstetrics and gynecology, worked with 19 premenopausal women who were being treated for benign uterine fibroids. (In doing medical research, large samples are nice, but you can't always get them, so you have to learn what you can from what's available. After all, you can't go into your local benign-uterine-fibroid bank and withdraw a thousand women.) The women took Lupron, which blocks the release of oestrogen from the ovaries, every four weeks for twelve weeks. They were then randomly assigned to receive either add-back oestrogen or placebo injections weekly for an additional eight weeks. When they were on Lupron, their scores on tests of verbal memory decreased from pretreatment to twelve weeks posttreatment, but those memory deficits were then reversed in the group that received oestrogen. These findings "strongly suggest that oestrogen serves to maintain verbal memory in women," the researchers concluded. Add-back oestrogen regimens may be important for maintaining memory in women being treated with oestrogen-suppressing medication as well as for women after menopause.[37]

And then there are the many studies that have followed women over even longer periods to see how they fared with and without oestrogen. The Cache County (Utah) study followed 2,114 women, average age 75 and all dementia-free at the start of the investigation, for twelve years. Their cognitive abilities were assessed every few years. The longer the women had been on oestrogen (on its own or as HRT), the better their cognitive status, and women who started taking hormones within 5 years of menopause had higher scores than those who began hormone therapy later.[38] In another study of 8,877 women in a retirement community followed for up to 14 years, oestrogen users had a 45 percent decreased risk of developing Alzheimer's disease.[39]

Ming-Xin Tang, a biostatistician in the Alzheimer's Disease Research Center at Columbia University, and his colleagues followed 1,124 older women (their average age was 74), initially free of Alzheimer's disease, who were taking part in a longitudinal study of aging and health in a New York City community. The researchers controlled for ethnicity, age, education, and APOE4 mutations. This was an observational study—meaning the women were not randomly assigned to take oestrogen or a placebo—but the results were highly suggestive: Among women taking oestrogen, the risk of developing Alzheimer's disease was significantly reduced by more than 60 percent; only 5.8 percent of the women on oestrogen (9 of 156) developed the disease, as compared to 16.3 percent of the women who were not taking oestrogen (158 of the 968). In addition, the age of onset of Alzheimer's disease occurred much later in women who were taking oestrogen than in those who were not.[40] These results have been replicated in many different locations around the world. An Italian study of 2,816 women found that oestrogen users had a 70 percent decreased risk of Alzheimer's disease.[41] And the large-scale Denmark PERF study (for "Prospective Epidemiological Risk Factors") found that women randomly assigned to take HRT for two to three years had a 64 percent decreased risk of cognitive impairment five to fifteen years later as compared with those on placebo who had never taken hormones.[42]

Across these studies and others, the percentages of the decreased risk of dementia and Alzheimer's vary quite a bit, from 24 percent to 70 percent. But they all point in the same general direction: that oestrogen helps. In 2000 and 2001, shortly before the first publication from the Women's Health Initiative, and in 2011, three large meta-analyses of existing studies concluded that overall, hormone replacement therapy was associated with a 34 percent decreased risk of dementia and a nearly 40 percent decrease in the risk of Alzheimer's.[43]

DOES OESTROGEN INCREASE THE RISK OF STROKE?

Another form of cognitive impairment that is deeply frightening comes from having a stroke; the decreased blood supply to the brain results in the loss of functioning brain tissue. For decades, it has been known that premenopausal women have a lower risk of stroke than men of the same age and that after menopause, women's annual risk of stroke increases exponentially. That protection is also reduced among women who are deprived of oestrogen before menopause.

We have noted that good observational studies often yield the same results as randomized controlled trials, but not always. Our goal for any given medical concern is to identify the overall picture that emerges from a variety of approaches, so let's see what that picture is for the risk of stroke for postmenopausal women who are taking HRT. Early observational studies produced a mixed bag of results. In some, HRT decreased the risk of stroke;[44] in some, HRT had no effect at all;[45] and in some, HRT increased the risk.[46] One factor that might affect those outcomes is whether women have cardiovascular disease when they begin taking hormones. Fortunately, two randomized controlled trials helped answer that question. In the first, 2,763 women with known heart disease, whose mean age at the beginning was 67, were followed for an average of 4 years. Those on HRT had no increased risk of stroke.[47] In the second, 664 women with a mean age of 71 at the outset and a history of prior stroke were followed for an average of nearly 3 years. The women treated with oestrogen alone and those treated with placebo did not differ in their risk of stroke.[48]

And then, in 2004, Garnet Anderson and the rest of the small WHI steering committee announced that the oestrogen-only arm of the study was being stopped because the use of oestrogen increased the risk of nonfatal stroke by 12 per 10,000 women per year.[49] This was precisely what they had reported in 2002, but apparently they didn't worry about it then; they waited 2 years to sound another alarm and set in motion another burst of "We're stopping the study!" headlines. Almost immediately, independent investigators strongly disputed this decision. Kate Maclaran and John Stevenson at the National Heart and Lung Institute, Imperial College London,[50] observed that the steering committee's concerns about stroke risks did not come at the recommendation of the WHI's own data safety and monitoring board. It was generated by the same inner group that had previously sounded the (false) alarm about hormones and breast cancer.

In fact, the WHI group had found no increase in any kind of serious stroke that led to incapacitation or death. They instead used an extremely broad definition of *stroke*—including transient, "subtle neurological deficits" that went away in a day or two with no aftermath. Some epidemiologists argued that this small apparent increase was artificially introduced by a "detection bias"—that is, the fact that women on HRT, having been made so sensitive to possible adverse effects of hormones after 2002, were hyperalert to any neurological symptoms. For example, if we told you that a tiny pimple on your forehead could indicate infection by a dangerous parasite, you'd become *very* attentive to tiny pimples. A team of physicians in Greece reanalyzed the WHI findings about the alleged risk of stroke, controlling for detection bias and the statistical manipulations that had appeared to indicate danger. The supposed increased risk of stroke vanished. Their paper, which appeared in the *Annals of the New York Academy of Sciences,* was titled "Pitfalls of the Women's Health Initiative." Far from supporting the WHI's decision to stop the study, these researchers concluded that "the use of HRT for 5 years should not be considered deleterious for the appearance of breast cancer, cardiovascular diseases, strokes, and pulmonary embolisms." The regimen should be individualized for each patient, they added, and, in the interest of caution, women with a family history of breast cancer, diagnosed coronary disease, or a predisposition to deep vein thromboses should have more intense follow-up to look for worsening of any of these potential complications.[51]

Likewise, Stanley Birge, a specialist in geriatric medicine, lamented the position of some medical societies that "persist in advising against the use of hormone therapy for the prevention of cardiovascular disease and osteoporosis" on the grounds that hormones increase the risk of stroke. That recommendation was ill-advised, he noted, because it was based on a misinterpretation of the WHI's data. The initial blip of increased risk among women most likely occurred because they were over 60, overweight, hypertensive, and smokers, and thus probably had some degree of atherosclerotic disease to begin with. For women like them, Birge concluded, taking hormones might in fact create a slightly elevated risk during the first two or three years of use. But, he added, "there was no risk of adverse outcomes five or more years after initiation of hormone therapy and [in] younger women without [preexisting vascular] disease."[52]

One further note: A 2015 Cochrane analysis found no increased risk of stroke among women who started taking hormones before age 60.[53] Cochrane reports are considered among the most reputable research findings in the medical literature, because they are meant to be impartial, independent assessments of the medical issue in question. (Archie Cochrane was a British physician who worked with Austin Bradford Hill and in 1972 wrote an influential book on the importance of evidence in medicine.) In a database of

RCTs of women given hormone therapy or placebo and followed for at least six months—a total of 19 trials with more than 40,000 women—women who started hormone therapy less than ten years after menopause had *fewer deaths* from cardiovascular causes and *lower rates* of coronary heart disease than women on placebo or no treatment. The Cochrane scientists concluded that there was "no strong evidence of effect on risk of stroke in this group."

Yet the Cochrane report issued one finding that is the reason that many doctors today still worry about the risk of stroke in *all* women on HRT: "an increased risk of stroke among women who started taking hormones more than 10 years after menopause." How did that "increased risk of stroke" get in there? A Cochrane report is only as good as the data it is based on, and this finding was heavily influenced by the largest RCT in the literature, the Women's Health Initiative.

RECONCILING THE EVIDENCE: THE OPTIMAL WINDOW

Today, most of the leading scientists who study oestrogen and brain function have refined the issue. Just as they concluded in assessing the risks and benefits of oestrogen for heart disease, they suggest that the questions to ask are no longer *whether* oestrogen helps but *whom* it helps and *when* it helps.

We have already mentioned one such investigator, Roberta Diaz Brinton, who summarized her view this way: For the most part, women who begin oestrogen or HRT at the time of menopause reduce their risk of getting many forms of dementia, including Alzheimer's.

But studies of women who are given oestrogen as a treatment —
once they have already developed a degree of dementia — have
mixed results. Among 5,500 patients who were followed at Kaiser
Permanente, women who had started taking hormones around
menopause had a 26 percent decreased risk of subsequent dementia, but those who started hormones many years after menopause
had a 48 percent increased risk.[54] Brinton concluded that "as the
continuum of neurological health progresses from healthy to
unhealthy, so too do the benefits of oestrogen or hormone therapy.
If neurons are healthy at the time of oestrogen exposure, their
response to oestrogen is beneficial for both neurological function
and survival."[55] But if those neurons are not healthy when a woman
starts oestrogen or if she begins taking HRT ten or more years after
menopause, oestrogen may, over time, make her condition worse.

Barbara Sherwin concluded too that the evidence from basic
neuroscience, from animal studies, and from human studies provided a strong case for a "critical window of opportunity." Oestrogen replacement in older women prevents some aspects of cognition
from deteriorating, as would occur with normal aging, she wrote,
and oestrogen "prevents or delays the onset of Alzheimer's disease
in women who are at risk for genetic or environmental reasons."[56]
But, she added, there is no evidence that oestrogen can slow or alleviate the disease once a woman has been diagnosed with it. Women
who start oestrogen when menopause begins, Sherwin said, thereby
"seamlessly extending" the number of years their brains are exposed
to it, will likely have less cognitive decline as they get older. Once
they stopped taking oestrogen, however, it was not clear whether its
protective benefits would continue into very old age; there were just
not enough good studies done with women that extended for thirty

years after menopause to know for sure, nor was such a large RCT ever likely to be done. Sherwin hoped that animal studies and "creative ways of asking this question in humans will provide some answers in the future."[57]

Pauline Maki has also proposed the window-of-opportunity hypothesis to reconcile the WHI's claims with the many studies that contradict it. Studies that reported an improvement in cognitive function, she observed, had assessed women who received oestrogen at the time of menopause, whereas those studies that reported no improvement, such as the Women's Health Initiative, involved women who started HRT many years after menopause. Women who started HRT somewhere between the ages of 50 and their early sixties had the greatest benefit; for women who began HRT in their sixties, hormones neither increased nor decreased their risk of Alzheimer's. A study whose name is hard to forget—the REMEM-BER study (from Research into Memory, Brain Function and Oestrogen Replacement)—likewise showed that the timing of hormone therapy for women over age 60 was important in determining whether oestrogen would help their later cognitive abilities.[58]

WHAT ABOUT THE ALTERNATIVES?

Most Americans don't like the idea that there are no drugs available to slow, let alone cure, Alzheimer's and other dementias, and this discomfort makes them vulnerable to the simplistic allures of untested products and promises. In 2017, the Federal Trade Commission filed a complaint against the makers of a bestselling supplement called Prevagen, claiming the company was falsely advertising it as a memory booster that gets "into the brain" and improves cognition. Prevagen, reportedly made from a protein in jellyfish, has been heavily marketed with commercials on CNN, Fox News, NBC, and elsewhere, mostly on the grounds that it is a bestselling product. "The marketers of Prevagen preyed on the fears of older consumers experiencing age-related memory loss," said the director of the FTC's Bureau of Consumer Protection. "But one critical thing these marketers forgot is that their claims need to be backed up by real scientific evidence."[59] There is none. In 2020, the makers of Prevagen settled a class action lawsuit with the FTC that required them to provide a disclaimer stating that the drug's effectiveness was "based on a clinical study of subgroups of individuals who were cognitively normal or mildly impaired." Don't buy it. The disclaimer or the drug.[60]

The many widely prescribed medications designed to prevent or slow the progress of Alzheimer's disease allow patients, physicians, and family members the comfort of thinking that *something* is being done, but sadly, those somethings are often no better than nothing, and they can quickly deplete a family's resources. But drug companies keep trying. The FDA has approved donepezil (Aricept), mirtazapine (Remeron), tacrine (Cognex, which was discontinued in the United States because of its link with liver damage), galantamine (Razadyne, formerly known as Reminyl), rivastigmine (Exelon), memantine (Ebixa or Namenda), and Namzaric, which combines donepezil and memantine. None of them have any effect on the progression of the disease. In 2018, *JAMA* published the unhappy results of three international randomized clinical trials of yet another drug, idalopirdine, summarized as another "therapeutic failure."[61]

The hottest recent drugs for treating Alzheimer's—aducanumab (Aduhelm), lecanemab (Leqembi), and gantenerumab—are antibodies directed against amyloid deposits in the brain. Unfortunately, as we said earlier, we do not yet know whether amyloid is a cause of, a contributor to, or simply a manifestation of the disease. To complicate matters, 14 percent of patients with Alzheimer's and over 30 percent of those with mild cognitive impairment test negative for the presence of amyloid. In any event, all three drugs have thus far yielded disappointing results.[62]

In 2023 a congressional committee slammed the FDA and the drug company Biogen for approving Aduhelm because of its lack of proven effectiveness and its outrageously high cost (more than $56,000 a year). Medicare eventually declined to cover Aduhelm and in 2024 Biogen discontinued testing and marketing it. The company reported that they planned to give up their ownership rights but added that they were not doing so "because of any concerns about the drug's safety or effectiveness." How reassuring. Leqembi has so far shown little real-life clinical benefit for people with dementia, and it has many serious side effects, including brain bleeding. (At least it costs "only" $26,500.) Gantenerumab's trials have failed to slow cognitive decline in people with early Alzheimer's. An editorial on its failure noted that "the results of the antibody trials to date either reinforce confidence in this therapeutic approach and its clinical meaningfulness or support a view that the effects are small, unreliable, and barely distinguishable from no effect."[63] We assume the results "reinforce confidence" for the drug manufacturer. Everyone else should take note of those small, unreliable, and barely detectable outcomes.

Unfortunately, sexism in research has been and still is alive and well in studies of these drugs. Although Alzheimer's disease is twice as common in women than men, the studies for the drugs have largely been done with men, and even when women and men are both in the study, the results are not evaluated separately.[64]

If not medication, what, then, might help?

Popular writers advise all kinds of benign interventions: eating a diet rich in antioxidants, reducing stress, engaging in stimulating mental activities like crossword puzzles, and exercising regularly. On the Mayo Clinic website, you'll find more of this optimistic all-purpose advice: "Regular exercise and a walking program have been found to prevent cognitive decline." That adviser apparently didn't speak to another physician on the website who answered the question "Are there any proven Alzheimer's prevention strategies?" with "Not yet."[65] While acknowledging that "more research is needed" before any advice could be considered a proven strategy, he added the usual recommendations to lead a healthy lifestyle: Get regular physical activity, preferably aerobic. Eat a healthy Mediterranean diet that is rich in vegetables and olive oil. Keep your brain active (all those crossword puzzles). Don't smoke. Control your blood pressure and cholesterol. Use your thinking skills. ("Use it or lose it" is a popular refrain, although gerontologists often gloomily add, "If you've lost it, you can't use it.")

We have no objection to healthy diets, olive oil, and exercise, mental and physical. But as interventions that might truly have a beneficial effect on delaying or averting cognitive decline and dementia in a woman's later years, compared to oestrogen, they don't do much.

Nowadays people are exhorted to regard the brain as just another muscle, one that can be exercised to keep it from getting flabby and plump. Memory exercises are today's mental weights; accordingly, numerous online programs are available to help people strengthen working memory, one of the mental systems responsible for storing and manipulating information. Working-memory training originated in 1999, when cognitive neuroscientist Torkel Klingberg created a computer program designed to help children with ADHD learn to focus. By 2001, he launched his company, Cogmed, and initial studies of children with attention deficit problems were promising. Naturally, that early success led to the hope that it would help people with other impairments of working memory—everything from mild learning difficulties to strokes and other forms of brain damage—improve their reasoning, everyday lapses of attention, and recall.

We're unhappy that we don't have happier news. One major meta-analysis of 87 working-memory training studies[66]—all of which were designed to see whether working-memory training helped short-term recall and if it transferred to other measures of mental ability—showed that typically, right after training, people improved on measures of near transfer—that is, doing what they had just learned to do. Practice doing puzzles and you get better at doing puzzles. Unfortunately, for measures of far transfer (nonverbal ability, verbal ability, word decoding, reading comprehension, and arithmetic), the researchers found "no convincing evidence of any reliable improvements when working-memory training was compared with a treated control condition.... Working-memory training programs appear to produce short-term, specific training effects that do not generalize to measures of 'real-world' cognitive skills." Damn.

At the Georgia Institute of Technology, memory scientist Randall W. Engel and his lab have discovered the same thing. In their own meta-analytic review, they concluded that "there is no good evidence that working-memory training improves intelligence test scores or other measures of 'real-world' cognitive skills."[67] Thomas Redick, another cognitive psychologist in their lab, took a close look at five studies that claimed to have demonstrated benefits of working-memory training; where benefits occurred right after the intervention, they were gone in a few months.[68] These findings were extended and confirmed in a 2016 meta-analysis of studies of "brain-training programs" that specifically focused on whether using cognitive tasks or games enhanced performance on other tasks.[69] Regrettably, they did not.

Okay, forget mental training, then; how about brain training? Transcranial direct-current stimulation (tDCS) — a noninvasive technique that applies electric current to areas of the brain — is growing in popularity for treating a variety of problems and disorders, from reducing depression to improving cognitive abilities. But applying tDCS to the brains of older people while they were immersed in working-memory training did not do much of anything for them. Researchers at the Karolinska Institute in Stockholm enrolled 123 healthy adults between the ages of 65 and 75 in a four-week training program. Everyone took a battery of cognitive tests at the beginning of the study and again at the end. Some participants received 25 minutes of tDCS to an area of the prefrontal cortex that plays a central role in working memory; others were led to believe they were receiving 25 minutes of current when in reality the current was active for only 30 seconds. The former group had no improvement in cognitive skills over their peers who got the sham treatment. When the researchers pooled the data from this study with findings from six other studies, they again saw no evidence of any additional benefit from working-memory training that was combined with tDCS.

The hope that tDCS would be a safe and effective way to improve cognitive function, the researchers concluded, "has been as seductive to the research community as it has been to the media. A growing number of people in the general public, presumably inspired by such uninhibited optimism, are now using tDCS to perform better at work or in online gaming, and online communities offer advice on the purchase, fabrication, and use of tDCS devices. Unsurprisingly, commercial exploitation is rapidly being developed to meet this new public demand for cognitive enhancement via tDCS, often without a single human trial to support the sellers' or manufacturers' claims."[70]

If mental exercises don't help memory and other cognitive abilities, how about physical exercise, which is widely believed to be an effective preventive for dementia? Notice the waffling tone in the Mayo Clinic's advice: "More research is needed to know to what degree adding physical activity improves memory or slows the progression of cognitive decline. Nonetheless, regular exercise is important to stay physically and mentally fit." Translation: Exercise is good, and it seems logical that it would slow the progression of cognitive decline and do other good things for your brain, but we don't yet know how much exercise or what kind is helpful. Still, do it anyway.

We agree, which is why we scoured the literature for evidence that exercise would keep our brains from declining any more than they have. There are literally hundreds of studies that claim to show that exercise helps forestall cognitive decline, but even the ten best ones disintegrate under close inspection. Some authors cite others' claims, not their own original research. Some rely on participants' memories of how much exercise they think they did—or remember thinking they did—years earlier, but self-reporting is notoriously unreliable. Some use measures of exercise that vary widely in both frequency (from one hour a week to one hour or more daily) and degree of intensity (from just getting out of your chair to vigorous walking or running). Or exercise is confounded with other risk factors, notably obesity, diabetes, lower education, and depression. And if exercise is difficult to measure accurately in these studies, so is cognitive decline; the measurements range from mild to severe. These complexities do not stop the writers of what we call "if-only" headlines, such as this one from the British paper the *Telegraph* purporting to summarize a new study: "One Hour of Exercise a Week 'Can Halve Dementia Risk.'" If only!

But because animal studies show that exercise does have neurological and vascular benefits in the brain, the effort to link those changes to cognitive abilities continues. In a meta-analysis of 47 longitudinal studies that tracked the effects of physical activity on cognitive decline and dementia, people with higher levels of physical activity were at reduced risk of cognitive decline, compared to those who were sedentary. What was that reduced risk? Only 18 percent. (Not to be sneezed at, though—get out of that chair.) Unfortunately, the better the study, the weaker the finding.[71] Another meta-analysis of 32 trials assessed the effectiveness of physical activity in slowing cognitive decline and delaying the onset of cognitive impairment and dementia among healthy adults. "The evidence was insufficient to draw conclusions about the effectiveness of aerobic training, resistance training, or tai chi for improving cognition," the researchers woefully concluded. Some interventions were helpful, but "evidence regarding effects on dementia prevention was insufficient for all physical activity interventions."[72]

The Take-Home

When Barbara Sherwin launched what would be her decades-long work on menopause, hormones, and memory, she feared the media might turn her findings into simplistic advice or, worse, use them to foster the misogynistic view of postmenopausal women's reduced cognitive abilities. Still, as she told a reporter at her home university of McGill, her goal has always been to help women live as enjoyably and productively as possible, and so she has little patience for those who dismiss HRT because it is "unnatural." "What's not natural is to live to 80," she said. Women live anywhere from one-third to one-half of their lives after menopause, and if oestrogen helps cognition and staves off Alzheimer's, that is crucial information. But "enhancing quality of life," she added, "is not the same as getting rid of the phenomenon of aging."[73]

In sum, there are good reasons to believe that oestrogen helps maintain cognitive abilities, along with preventing cardiovascular disease and stroke. To review:

- Oestrogen stimulates the growth of nerve cells, regenerates axons, and decreases the nerve-cell death that happens in Alzheimer's.
- Oestrogen reduces levels of vasoconstrictors, substances that narrow the arteries; increases levels of vasodilators, substances that expand them; increases cerebral blood flow; and inhibits inflammatory substances that are involved in the early stages of atherosclerosis.
- Oestrogen enhances the ability of neurons to survive a variety of physiological insults, such as disease and brain injury.

But what about the Women's Health Initiative and its history of scaring women?

- The WHI did not find an increased risk of dementia or cognitive impairment in women on oestrogen only. On the contrary, oestrogen alone significantly decreased the risk of dementia when started at midlife (around 45 to 54 years of age).
- The risk of dementia was slightly increased among women on HRT, but only if they had preexisting cognitive impairments or were starting hormones long past menopause.
- The WHI did not find that oestrogen increased the risk of stroke in younger women entering menopause who were in good vascular health. There was an increased risk in women who were over 60, overweight, hypertensive, and smokers, and thus probably had some degree of atherosclerotic disease to begin with.
- The WHI, as usual, made a lot of noise about HRT's harms (dementia! stroke!) but buried HRT's benefits. The WHI's own data showed that women who had taken hormones prior to entering the study and therefore closer to the time of menopause were less likely to develop all forms of dementia, including Alzheimer's, during the clinical trial. They had a reduction of risk of 50 percent compared to nonusers.[74]

Bottom line: Just as with oestrogen's benefits for heart and bones, there does seem to be a window of opportunity for oestrogen to have a long-standing cognitive benefit: the decade following the onset of menopause. If oestrogen is begun after around age 65 or many years after menopause begins, it may be ineffective and possibly risky.

This conclusion was supported in the biggest meta-analysis to date of the research on hormones and dementia, published in 2023 in *Frontiers in Aging Neuroscience*. The fifteen authors, who include Roberta Diaz Brinton and Lisa Mosconi (leading scientists whose work we have already mentioned in this chapter), reviewed six RCTs (about 21,000 women on hormones and a comparable number on placebo) and 45 observational studies (involving 768,866 women on hormones and 5.5 million controls).[75] Their conclusions were appropriately cautious, because so many factors are involved in trying to determine whether hormones started in a woman's early fifties affect her risk of dementia twenty or thirty years later. That's why some studies have found a benefit, some have found a small risk, and some have found neither benefit nor risk.

So what's a woman to do? The clearest finding in their review paper was this: The RCT results showed a small increased risk for postmenopausal women who were over age 65 when they began combination HRT. You know which study was largely responsible for that conclusion, don't you? (Clue: its acronym is WHI.) Here we go again: "Late-life [hormone therapy] use was associated with increased risk, albeit not significant."

But wait, you say—what about that scary Danish study mentioned earlier, the one that made headlines everywhere and claimed to find a connection between HRT and cognitive decline?[76] Have you been paying attention to what we keep saying is usually wrong with alarmist headlines? That "connection" is not what the study demonstrated. The authors collected menopausal hormone prescription data on 5,589 women ages 50 to 60 and who had developed dementia between 2000 and 2018. They collected similar data on 55,890 women in the same age range who had not developed dementia during those years. So this was not a study in which women were randomly assigned to hormones or no hormones and then followed over time; the researchers simply combed through the retrospective data they collected in search of possible correlations. And what did they find?

- *No* increased risk of dementia among women taking only oestrogen.
- *No* increased risk of dementia among women taking only progesterone.
- A small but statistically significant increased risk of dementia among users of combined oestrogen-progesterone. How did the groups differ? Trivially: 31.9 percent of the dementia patients had taken HRT, while 28.9 percent of the control patients who didn't develop dementia had taken this same combination in the past.

The two groups took hormones for close to the same length of time: 3.8 years for the dementia group and 3.6 years for controls. (Really? A couple of months on hormones is enough to increase your risk of dementia?) Further, the researchers did not determine whether these women had family histories of dementia, even though that factor would significantly affect the results.

So bad was this "study" that a senior investigator from the WHI, a coauthor of an editorial critiquing it, observed that dementia risk with less than one year of hormone treatment was not biologically plausible.[77] The researchers did not even cite the PERF study by their own fellow Danes (see p. 192) that showed that women randomly assigned to take HRT for 2 to 3 years had a 64 percent *decreased* risk of cognitive impairment 5 to 15 years later compared with those who had never taken HRT.[78]

*   *   *

Among the many messages that Avrum has received over the years, one email, from a frustrated, angry former patient we'll call Linda, summarizes the struggles of countless women today. Nearly twenty-five years ago, she had had an invasive breast cancer that was greater than two centimeters; her lymph nodes were negative for cancer, and she was treated with a lumpectomy, radiation, and chemotherapy. She had been on Premarin and progesterone ever since and had had no evidence of recurrence in all those years. After she moved out of state, she wrote to Av: "I'm still taking HRT and would appreciate getting a copy of your pertinent research on it because I have to beg the doctors to approve it or prescribe it. I once stopped it, but within two or three weeks I became very old and couldn't remember a thing. I was in a meeting and at some point I realized I had just asked the same question for the third time. Imagine my embarrassment! I've never stopped [HRT] again."

When Albert Einstein was asked what he considered his major scientific talent, he said it was his ability to look at a large number of experiments, select those that were correct, ignore the rest, and build a theory on the right ones. It does not take the genius of Einstein to conclude that the Danish study and the familiar, overblown alarms from the WHI should be ignored. Avrum sent Linda the information in this chapter, and we hope that it persuaded Linda's doctor . . . as it has persuaded us.

7

Progesterone and the Pill

Dear Dr. Bluming:

I know for me, personally, the dilemma is no longer about taking oestrogen, but rather about what to do concerning progesterone, which seems to have become the new villain. I've even contemplated having my uterus removed so as not to have to take progesterone and not subject myself to all its downsides, although that feels ridiculously radical to me.

Yes, it certainly is! Over the years, whenever Avrum has written or lectured about the benefits of HRT and the misconceptions about the harms of oestrogen, he is often asked two "what-about" questions:

What about progesterone? What about birth control pills?

"My daughter is on the pill," wrote an older woman, "but I

remember the early days when the pill had very high oestrogen levels and I've been suspicious about it ever since. Should I worry? Does the pill increase her risk of breast cancer?"

To answer these concerns, let's look at the evidence.

WHAT ABOUT PROGESTERONE?

Progesterone was isolated and purified in the early 1930s by scientists in several countries who together agreed to call it *progesterone* because it is the hormone that supports pregnancy (*pro*-gestation). Progesterone stimulates the cells in the uterine lining to proliferate in preparation for the possible arrival of a fertilized egg. The level of circulating progesterone increases during the latter half of the menstrual cycle but declines back to its resting level if fertilization does not occur. If it does, the level of progesterone continues to rise, stimulating the endometrial cells to provide a nourishing environment for the fetus.

Today, the word *progesterone* is often misleadingly applied to a variety of related but different preparations. In the United States, the most commonly used natural form is micronized progesterone, sold as Prometrium. In contrast, *progestins* are synthetic compounds that mimic the activity of progesterone. The most frequently prescribed progestin is medroxyprogesterone acetate (MPA, sold as Provera). Prempro, a common form of hormone replacement therapy, is a combination of oestrogen and MPA; this was the HRT used in the Women's Health Initiative study.

We can answer Av's first questioner right off the bat: Keep your uterus and take the progesterone. But she was right to observe that progesterone "seems to have become the new villain." The WHI's study in 2002 reported that oestrogen on its own did not increase the risk of breast cancer; in fact, as we have seen, over the ensuing years in which they did follow-ups, it was associated with a decreased risk.[1] As one researcher summarized: "The only statistically significant outcome for all participants (50–79 years) in the WHI Oestrogen-Alone Trial for the 13-year cumulative long-term follow-up was a reduction in invasive breast cancer with CEE [Premarin]."[2]

And so, to continue making the case against HRT, the WHI investigators and their supporters argued that it was the addition of progesterone that was harmful.[3] Once again, however, considerable evidence exonerates progesterone. Women who have a progesterone deficiency—because they fail to ovulate or for some other reason—have a higher risk of developing breast cancer; in one study of more than a thousand premenopausal women with progesterone deficiency, the risk was five times as high.[4] In addition, as with oestrogen, progesterone is often used as a treatment for breast cancer:

- A prospective, randomized study of postmenopausal women with advanced breast cancer found that 44 percent of those treated with MPA had partial or complete remission, compared to 35 percent of the women treated with tamoxifen. In fact, MPA was even more effective than tamoxifen in the treatment of bone metastases and for women over 70. A subsequent review of all randomized clinical trials comparing tamoxifen with progestins for metastatic breast cancer in postmenopausal women confirmed these findings.[5]
- In a randomized controlled trial of a thousand women about to have surgery for breast cancer, a surgical oncologist in

Mumbai, India, injected half of them with a single dose of progesterone five to fourteen days before operating. Five years later, this injection had significantly improved the disease-free prognosis for women who had positive node involvement compared to those who did not receive the progesterone.[6] (The women with no lymph-node involvement already had a favorable prognosis.)

- In a study of 4,575 women ages 35 to 64 who had survived invasive breast cancer, those who had been taking progestin-only contraceptives for four years did not have an increased risk of cancer recurrence compared with a control group.[7]

Progesterone may improve breast cancer survival rates. Australian scientists found that receptors that mediate the activity of oestrogen and progesterone interact with DNA to control the growth of a large majority of breast cancers. Their discovery may bode well for targeted treatments. A team at the University of Cambridge's Cancer Research UK Institute reported that natural progesterone can stimulate the progesterone receptor on a breast cancer cell, resulting in suppression of its growth.[8]

Perhaps, then, it's not the natural, purer forms of progesterone that are the problem so much as progestins, the synthetic versions that were used in the Women's Health Initiative. Guess who promoted that idea? Right. The data linking the combination of oestrogen and progestin to an increased risk of breast cancer came largely from the WHI, whose own findings on this matter, as we saw in chapters 2 and 3, were barely statistically significant and inconsistent across their follow-up reports.

Indeed, some investigators have argued that the WHI did not find a true increased risk but a statistically spurious one.[9] Richard Santen, an endocrinologist and professor of medicine at the University of Virginia, and his colleagues put the matter in perspective. They themselves do not think HRT should be taken for more than a few years because of its presumed risks of breast cancer, but they acknowledged that the risk is low. "Based on the worst-case analysis," they wrote, "...women taking HRT for 10 [years] have a 96% chance of remaining free of breast cancer vs. 98% of those not taking HRT."[10] It is still not known why progestins should have a slightly higher risk than progesterone. Some progestins stimulate androgen receptors (which both women and men have, though obviously in different proportions). High levels of free testosterone (an androgen) have been identified as a risk factor in breast cancer both before and after menopause.[11] Italian researchers removed the ovaries of adult female monkeys and then randomly assigned them to be given oestrogen plus progestin or a placebo. The monkeys on the progestin developed a greater proliferation of the single layer of epithelial cells that line the breast's milk ducts. When the monkeys were put on micronized (natural) progesterone instead of progestin, no increased proliferation of cells occurred.[12] Again, the precise biological mechanism behind this result is unclear, but perhaps one reason is that micronized progesterone does not stimulate androgen receptors as progestins do. In 2005, an extensive literature review by another Italian group concluded that using oral micronized progesterone eliminated any increased risk of breast cancer associated with HRT.[13]

Don't throw out your Provera just yet! It might seem from these studies that women who wish to be on HRT should, to feel safest, take progesterone in its oral, micronized form. Yet even so, we are talking about extremely small differences in risks between progesterone and progestin—no more than a 2 percent bump. Some women, including Av's wife, Martha, do better in terms of side effects with Provera (the progestin) than with micronized progesterone, and they should not be unduly concerned. And remember that even if HRT with progestin increases the risk of breast cancer by a tiny percentage, we have bombarded you with evidence that women on HRT live longer and have a lower death rate from breast cancer than those who are not on HRT.

There's one other important consideration to keep in mind about the benefits of HRT: It appreciably reduces the risk of colon cancer, the third most common cancer in the United States. In 2023, the projections were that there would be more than 150,000 new cases every year and about one-third of those patients would die.[14] However, the rate of colon cancer is consistently lower for women, especially premenopausal women who are producing their own oestrogen, suggesting that oestrogen protects against the growth of cancerous cells in the colon.[15] After menopause, women who take HRT have a lower risk of getting colon cancer and a lower mortality rate if they do get it compared with women not on hormones.[16] Not all studies have gotten these results,[17] but the preponderance of them have. Even the Women's Health Initiative did. In an analysis of all women enrolled in the WHI, the use of any form of HRT reduced the risk of colon cancer by 30 percent. In a similar study, both oestrogen alone and progestin plus oestrogen—in any form, patch or pill—were associated with a "strong reduction" in the risk of colon cancer.[18]

WHAT ABOUT BIRTH CONTROL PILLS?

The first oral contraceptive, Enovid, was approved in 1960, although it was illegal for unmarried women to use it (or any other birth control, for that matter) in 26 states. Five years later, in its landmark decision *Griswold v. Connecticut,* the Supreme Court ruled that it was unconstitutional for the government to prohibit married couples from using birth control. The court did not quite get up the nerve to legalize birth control for all American women until 1972, in *Eisenstadt v. Baird.*

The oestrogen most commonly used in birth control pills is ethinyl estradiol. In the early years, when the pill contained relatively high doses of oestrogen (Enovid had as much as 10 milligrams of ethinyl estradiol), a small but worrying number of women developed blood clots in their veins, usually in the legs. Sometimes, fragments of those clots broke off and traveled to the lungs, leading to pulmonary emboli and, in some cases, death.[19] This lethal complication was clearly unacceptable, and the shock of its occurring in otherwise healthy young women caused a national uproar. As a result, the dose of hormones in these pills was cut way down, and emboli are now extremely rare.[20]

In today's oral contraceptives, ethinyl estradiol comes in a variety of dosages. Some are higher than the dose used in HRT, and some are lower. Some low-dose oral contraceptives contain only 0.01 milligram of ethinyl estradiol and tend to be prescribed primarily for perimenopausal women who want contraception but who also have irregular or heavy menses or hormonally related symptoms that impair quality of life. These preparations provide adequate oestrogen to relieve hot flushes and other vasomotor symptoms.[21] (The progesterone components of birth control pills and HRT are often similar.)

At any of these doses, oral contraceptives are among the most effective birth control methods we have, with failure rates of less than 1 percent when used as directed. We also now have more than sixty years of research on their safety, and for women who are concerned about oestrogen and breast cancer, the findings are immensely reassuring—even for breast cancer survivors:

- Throughout the 1980s, a series of large-scale studies from the Centers for Disease Control's Cancer and Steroid Hormone (CASH) Study repeatedly found no significant association between oral contraceptive use and breast cancer, even when it was used at an early age, before first pregnancy, at the time of diagnosis, or in women with a family history of breast cancer.[22]
- In 2002, the CDC evaluated 4,574 women with breast cancer and 4,682 controls. More than 75 percent of these women were using or had used oral contraceptives. There was no increased risk of breast cancer associated with duration of use or age at which a woman began taking the pill (including those younger than 20).[23]
- In 2007, a large British cohort study of 46,000 women, half of whom took oral contraceptives and all of whom had been followed for an average of 24 years, found no difference in breast cancer incidence among users and never-users.[24]
- In 2008, the WECARE (Women's Environment, Cancer, and Radiation Epidemiology) study compared 708 women who had had cancer in both breasts with 1,395 women who

had had cancer in one breast and found that oral contraceptive use did not increase the risk of developing cancer in the opposite breast. Years on the pill made no difference and neither did age of starting it. A follow-up study of women with primary breast cancer who were also BRCA1 or BRCA2 mutation carriers again found no association between use of oral contraceptives and risk of breast cancer in the opposite breast.[25]

- In 2010, the Nurses' Health Study reported that among 1,344 breast cancer patients, only 57 women had a small increased risk of breast cancer. But this small increased risk was seen only among those who were taking a progestin known to stimulate androgen receptors. Because of the very low numbers, the authors concluded that "current oral contraceptive use is not a major cause of breast cancer."[26]

- In 2013, a meta-analysis of 13 prospective studies involving 11,722 cases of breast cancer among 850,000 women found no significant association between the use of oral contraceptives (past or present) and breast cancer.[27]

- As with other findings about oestrogen, survival rates for breast cancer patients tend to be higher in women taking oral contraceptives at the time of their diagnosis than in women not taking oestrogen.[28]

Here is some truly stunning news. The number of ovarian cancers diagnosed in the United States each year is small compared to the number of newly diagnosed breast cancers — 20,000 ovarian cancers compared to 240,000 breast cancers. Ovarian cancer is much more difficult to treat and cure; there's still no good screening test for it, and, in 2023, its mortality rate (67 percent) remained many times higher than that of newly diagnosed breast cancer.[29] Yet the available evidence suggests that oral contraceptives decrease the risk of ovarian cancer by 40 to 80 percent.[30] In one study, epidemiologist Martin Vessey and his colleague Rosemary Painter, in the department of public health at the University of Oxford, looked at more than 17,000 women recruited from family-planning clinics between 1968 and 1974 and followed until 2004. Women who had been taking oral contraceptives were 40 percent less likely to develop ovarian cancer than women who had never taken the pill. Moreover, women taking the pill for more than ten years reduced their overall risk of ovarian cancer by as much as 80 percent, and this benefit persisted for nearly twenty years after they stopped oral contraception.[31]

Epidemiological studies, whether of small or large populations, will never get 100 percent concordance in results. That's why we must look for the picture that emerges from the larger mosaic formed by all the pieces of evidence, even if a few don't fit. With the question of birth control pills and breast cancer, as usual, a few pieces don't fit, and those pieces — showing a small but significant increase in the risk of breast cancer among women taking oral contraceptives — should be noted.

In 1996, the Collaborative Group on Hormonal Factors in Breast Cancer performed a meta-analysis of 54 epidemiologic studies from around the world on oral contraceptive use and invasive breast cancer[32] — totaling 53,297 women with breast cancer and 100,239 women without breast cancer. Women taking oral contraceptives had a small increased risk of developing invasive breast cancer, a risk that remained for 10 years after stopping the pill. It was, however, a very small increased risk. How small? Small enough that in a subsequent review, the authors waved it away. Because rates of breast cancer among women young enough to be on birth control were so low, they said this time, and because the absolute numbers of women in the sample who developed breast cancer were, accordingly, very small, any apparent increase in breast cancer risk due to birth control pills was trivial.[33]

Nevertheless, as night follows day and penguins follow fish, scare stories will ever be upon us. They are...scary. They get our attention. They draw readers. They sell. We were not surprised when, in 2017, a friend called us to ask about a *New York Times* article that worried her. The headline was dramatic: "Birth Control Pills Still Linked to Breast Cancer, Study Finds," as was the subhead: "Women Using Birth Control Pills and I.U.D.s That Release Hormones Face a Higher Risk than Those Using Methods without Hormones, Scientists in Denmark Reported."[34] The article reported on a nationwide cohort study, published in the *New England Journal of Medicine,* involving 1.8 million Danish women between the ages of 15 and 49 who had been followed for 10 years. The researchers found an increase in breast cancers among current and recent users of oral contraceptives and in women using IUDs that released progestin.[35]

The *New York Times* reporter, Roni Caryn Rabin, noted right away that the "absolute risk was small." In fact, in an accompanying editorial in the *NEJM* titled "Oral Contraceptives and the Small Increased Risk of Breast Cancer," David J. Hunter, a professor of epidemiology and medicine at the University of Oxford, emphasized how small it was: "An increase of around one new breast cancer case per 7,690 current and recent users of hormonal contraception." He placed the findings in the context of previous research, including the studies that found an increased risk, such as the one from the Collaborative Group on Hormonal Factors in Breast Cancer, and those that did not, such as the Centers for Disease Control reports. He concluded, as the Collaborative Group had, that the clinical implications of this study "must be placed in the context of the low incidence rates of breast cancer among younger women," pointing out that most of the new breast cancer cases occurring in the study were among women over the age of 40 who were still on the pill. Most important, he wrote, "the risk of breast cancer needs to be balanced against the benefits of the use of oral contraceptives," and the risks were far outweighed by the pill's many impressive benefits: it provided effective contraception, helped women who have painful menstrual periods or abnormally heavy bleeding, and was associated with substantial reductions in the risks of ovarian, endometrial, and colorectal cancers later in life.[36]

As if to underscore the point, the reporter inserted a link smack in the middle of her story to an article titled "Birth Control Pills Protect Against Cancer, Too."

Indeed they do, as shown in a prospective analysis of more than 196,536 women, followed from 1995 to 2011. The researchers found a 40 percent reduction in the incidence of ovarian cancer in the women who had been taking oral contraceptives for at least ten years, and a similar reduction in the incidence of endometrial cancer. They found no association between oral contraception and the likelihood of developing breast cancer.[37]

And yet some investigators remain determined to scare women away from oestrogen. Over and over, they have inflated the tiniest statistics into the largest alarms. Valerie Beral was a lead author of the 1996 Collaborative Reanalysis, the study in which the researchers themselves waved away their finding of "increased risk" as trivial. She was also the lead author of the Million Women Study, which we criticized vigorously in the breast cancer chapters. In 2023, Valerie Beral and her colleagues published a meta-analysis, and it is no surprise that once again, they reported an increased risk of breast cancer among young women who had taken the pill for at least 5 years. There was no increased risk of death from breast cancer, and how serious was the increased risk of developing it? Eight cases per 100,000 users.[38]

The Take-Home

Because many women are concerned about the possible risks of progesterone and birth control pills, let's review:

- The word *progesterone*, the natural hormone that supports pregnancy (pro-gestation), is often applied to different preparations. The most commonly used natural form is micronized progesterone (Prometrium). In contrast, progestins are synthetic compounds that mimic the activity of progesterone. In the United States, the most frequently prescribed progestin is medroxyprogesterone acetate (MPA, sold as Provera).
- Although progesterone seems to have become a new villain in arguments against HRT, the preponderance of evidence exonerates it. As with oestrogen, progesterone is often used as an effective treatment for women with breast cancer and may even improve breast cancer survival rates.

- Investigators have reported no increased risk of breast cancer among women on HRT when the form of progesterone was oral (natural) micronized progesterone and a very small and debatable increase in risk—only 2 percent—when the progesterone was a synthetic progestin. Nonetheless, some women who take HRT do better with a progestin than with micronized progesterone. They should not be concerned because of the more important overall finding that women on HRT live longer and have a significantly lower death rate from breast cancer than those not taking HRT.

- Women on any formulation of oestrogen or HRT have a significant reduction in the risk of colon cancer.

- Oral contraceptives are overwhelmingly safe and highly effective. The vast majority of studies have found no association between use of oral contraceptives and breast cancer, and in those few that have, the finding is trivial. This holds regardless of how young a woman was when she began taking the pill, whether she used it before her first pregnancy, whether she was on the pill at the time of diagnosis, or whether she has a family history of breast cancer.

The challenge, researchers and physicians agree, is to neither ignore small risks nor inflate them into looming dangers. "Nothing is risk-free, and hormonal contraceptives are not an exception to that rule," Øjvind Lidegaard, one of the authors of the NEJM paper, told the New York Times.[39] As we have stressed repeatedly, every medical intervention, whether it is a diagnostic test, surgery, or medication, carries a risk. Even something that might seem entirely beneficial, such as taking vitamins, can have risk. How can vitamins be bad for you? An overdose of vitamin A or vitamin D can be lethal. Which risks should consumers take into consideration, and which are trivial? Most people who watch pharmaceutical ads on TV now tune out the obligatory warnings about side effects, which can include everything from rashes to death. The list is so long that it is comical, yet the warnings are deadly serious. Literally.

So consumers must find a path between regarding serious warnings as trivial and taking trivial warnings too seriously. That is why we are concerned that the FDA continues to require that black box warning on all oestrogen products, initiated so long ago in the wake of the WHI's alarms. All hormone therapy products, including vaginal creams with oestrogen, must have that warning to alert users to the "risks" of heart attacks, strokes, breast cancer, and dementia. In an editorial for the *Journal of the North American Menopause Society*, Cynthia Stuenkel wrote, "Many clinicians have experienced the dismay of prescribing vaginal oestrogen, only to have their patient return in follow-up with the news that after reading the patient package insert, she (or her partner) had decided not to chance the perils as highlighted in the boxed warning."[40] No wonder. Comfortable sex probably isn't worth a heart attack, cancer, or dementia!

But wonders never cease, and progress marches on. In January 2018, the Women's Health Initiative investigators announced that the dose of oestrogen in vaginal creams is not associated with an increased risk of breast cancer.[41] It took them only sixteen years, so who knows — maybe in another sixteen years, they will also change their minds about HRT.

Vaginal oestrogen is also safe for women with breast cancer. A

2024 study of nearly 50,000 breast cancer patients in Northern Ireland matched women using vaginal oestrogen with controls by age, stage of their cancer, and other factors. At the 8-year follow-up, the women using vaginal oestrogen had no increased risk of death from breast cancer. "This finding may provide some reassurance to prescribing physicians," the researchers concluded, "and support the guidelines suggesting that vaginal oestrogen therapy can be considered in patients with breast cancer and genitourinary symptoms."[42] Some reassurance to women too!

8

Debates and Final Lessons in the Case for HRT

I n this final chapter, Avrum will describe the challenge of finding common ground with colleagues who disagree with him,
review the benefits and risks of HRT, and answer some questions that his patients frequently ask him, questions that you may
have also. For readers whose physicians still closely adhere to guidelines informed by the Women's Health Initiative, Av provides a list
of its ten key problems in hopes that it will prove a useful start for
conversation.

*　　*　　*

Many years ago, I was invited to debate Susan Love, then the director of the UCLA Breast Center, on the topic of oestrogen and breast
cancer for an audience of physicians and cancer researchers in
Southern California. As the guest speaker, I was first. I started by

saying I felt sure that when the debate was over, everyone, including Susan, would have reached some point of agreement, because, after all, we had the same goal: the prevention and eradication of breast cancer. I presented my case, summarizing the gist of what you have read in this book, and then sat down to hear her response.

Love began by saying she would never agree with me because she objected strongly to the idea that menopause was a disease, and anyone who suggested that hormone replacement therapy had any benefits was clearly labeling menopause a disease that needed treatment. Girls did very well until they reached the age of puberty, she said, and then they spent the next several decades on a tumultuous emotional and physical roller coaster. Only after menopause, she said, did women finally have a chance to run companies, colleges, and countries and become political activists. The problem, Love concluded, wasn't that women suffered oestrogen deficiency following menopause; it was that they suffered "oestrogen poisoning" between puberty and menopause.

Her remarks were followed by dead silence.

Susan Love, who died in 2023, went on to become director of what is now the Dr. Susan Love Foundation for Breast Cancer Research, and she wrote many popular books. Among them is *Dr. Susan Love's Menopause and Hormone Book,* which repeats the oestrogen-poisoning line and lists the benefits of menopause; it is a time, she said, when women no longer feel "constrained by the dictates of finding a man for reproduction."[1] She continued to promote the view that the medicalization of menopause is bad for women, an unnecessary intrusion into a normal phase of women's lives.

Still, it was easier for me to debate Susan Love, whose position was clear if simplistic, than to debate, on separate occasions over the ensuing years, the eminent physicians and epidemiologists who either worked with the WHI, supported its primary claims, or were convinced that oestrogen was a carcinogen. One such expert is epidemiologist Malcolm Pike, who has a PhD in mathematical statistics and is a former director of the Cancer Epidemiology Unit at Oxford University, a former director of the USC epidemiology department, and currently attending epidemiologist at Memorial Sloan Kettering Cancer Center. Pike has long maintained that breast cancer *is* related to hormone levels, and by now you know why I believe that position, no matter how many prominent experts hold it, is unsupported by a vast number of disconfirming studies.

During my debate with Pike in 2003, in front of an audience of physicians attending a continuing medical education program, I sought common ground, as I always try to do. "We agree," I said to him, "that the incidence of breast cancer continues to rise through and past menopause, even in women who are not on HRT. If oestrogen were really a cause of breast cancer, shouldn't that rate decline — indeed, shouldn't it drop precipitously, given that levels of circulating oestrogen drop so sharply following menopause?" He agreed that rates of breast cancer continue to rise in older women as their oestrogen levels fall. But, he countered, the *rate of increase* slows as oestrogen drops.

I thought, *Pardon me?* Aloud I asked, "How does this bear on my argument? The point is that rates of breast cancer continue to rise steadily into old age. If oestrogen is a primary contributor to breast cancer, those rates should steadily decline. Why don't they?"

"I'm not a real doctor the way Dr. Bluming is," Pike joked to the audience. "All I have is a PhD, not an MD, but my PhD is in statistics"—the implication being that his possession of that degree was an adequate answer.

In 2007, I had the opportunity to debate Peter Ravdin, MD, PhD, on a radio show during the San Antonio Breast Cancer Symposium; we discussed the relation of HRT to breast cancer. Ravdin, director of the Breast Health Clinic at the University of Texas, later won a Pathfinder Award from the American Society of Breast Disease, celebrating him as "an innovator who has combined biological intuition, clinical and translational research, and clinical practice with an interdisciplinary understanding to advance the fight against breast disease and breast cancer." During our debate, Ravdin noted that the incidence of breast cancer declined within eight months after the first report of the Women's Health Initiative in 2002, and, for want of an alternative explanation, he attributed that decline to the fact that the number of HRT prescriptions had nose-dived and women were no longer taking that risky oestrogen-progestin combination.

If you read chapter 2, you know how I replied. "Unfortunately for that argument," I countered, "that decline started in 1999, long before the 2002 publication of the WHI. Moreover, most breast cancers take at least nine years to become diagnosable tumors— far longer than eight months."

Well, Ravdin said, actually he was talking about the very small, not-yet-diagnosed, "subclinical" cancers of the breast that, he conjectured, stopped growing when HRT was discontinued.[2]

"That isn't a credible position," I replied, "because the primary decrease is occurring in larger, invasive tumors, which take far longer to develop than eight months. Besides, there has been no decline in breast cancer rates among Black women or women in

Europe who went off hormones. Further, the overwhelming majority of women who take HRT do not develop breast cancer, and the overwhelming majority of women who do develop breast cancer do not take HRT—and you have no evidence that the decline occurred *only* among women who had been on HRT and stopped." I was warming to the challenge. "And by the way, in many European countries where women went off HRT following the Women's Health Initiative at the same rates as here, there was no decline in breast cancer. How, then, can you claim credit on behalf of the WHI for a decline in breast cancer rates in America but not elsewhere and only among white women?"

He had no reply except to repeat his conviction that the WHI had saved many lives by getting women off HRT. That year, when I and several other writers criticized the WHI in print for taking credit for the decline in breast cancer rates, Ravdin and his colleagues still maintained that "although there is no conclusive proof of a causal link between coincident sharp declines in the use of hormone-replacement therapy and the incidence of oestrogen-receptor-positive breast cancer, we have yet to see a credible alternative explanation."[3] What does that mean? It means we can't explain the decline in breast cancer rates, but we'll cheerfully take credit for it.

Malcolm Pike and Peter Ravdin are giants in their fields, deservedly honored. But their eminence should not blind us to the inherent contradiction in their arguments. Ravdin says that when oestrogen declines because women go off HRT, breast cancer declines. Pike says that when oestrogen declines as women age, breast cancer rates rise—but "at a slower rate." Both of these men were twisting the evidence to fit their preconceived beliefs.

I have been reading comments by the WHI investigators for

many years. Some individuals among them have dogmatically stuck to their original positions, still maintaining that the WHI was *the* very best study ever and therefore offers the most reliable evidence that HRT causes breast cancer. Others have cautiously admitted that maybe those early scare stories were, um, premature and a bit overblown. Others have conducted subsequent reanalyses that contradicted their earlier conclusions, but instead of conceding error, they typically waffle, unable to say a good word for HRT even when their own evidence shows that they can.

For example, by 2012, the WHI investigators were already backtracking on their claims about oestrogen and breast cancer. Women on oestrogen alone, they reported, were less likely to die of breast cancer—indeed, less likely to die from all causes after a breast cancer diagnosis—than women assigned to placebo.[4] Yet the report's lead author, Garnet Anderson, told the *Seattle Times* that "the results were not favorable for women with a family history of breast cancer" (untrue, as we saw earlier when we discussed the research on BRCA-positive women); that the "combination-pill trial, closed in 2002, found women taking Prempro...had a higher risk of breast cancer" (untrue; the risk was not statistically significant); that "the oestrogen-only trial, shut down in 2004, found a risk of stroke and no protection from heart attacks" (not accurate); and that "we can't say what would happen if these women stayed on oestrogen for 10 or 15 years" (yes, we can; we have ample data from the many studies of women who have taken hormones for 10, 15, and 20 years).[5]

What about their important finding of fewer deaths among women on oestrogen? Anderson advised caution because "the mortality data are thin." But those findings were statistically significant, and other studies support the conclusion that HRT prolongs women's lives. Yet she was satisfied enough with "thin data" when she and her fellow investigators could fatten them up to worry the public with nonsignificant claims that HRT increases the risk of death from all causes. She chose caution only when dealing with good news. On one of the most important findings from her own project—that when taken during the "window of benefit" after the onset of menopause, HRT confers protection against heart attacks and strokes—Anderson was silent. By the way, she is not a physician; she is a biostatistician.

Or consider JoAnn Manson's assessment in 2015, in which she wrote that while she still believed that HRT increased the risk of breast cancer, she was willing to agree that the risk was "offset" by the protection HRT affords against bone fractures, diabetes, and endometrial cancer. Seemingly having forgotten the WHI's early claim that HRT increases rates of "all-cause mortality," she said that it all balances out. "We can reassure women now," she told the *Times* (UK). "Even though there are risks, there are counterbalancing benefits that mean the effect on mortality is neutral."[6] In 2017, Manson and her colleagues reported that women who had taken oestrogen or HRT and had been followed for up to eighteen years had *no* extra deaths from heart disease, breast cancer, any other kind of cancer, or, for that matter, from any other disease compared to the control group.[7]

Where were the press releases and headlines saying "Sorry, everyone, that we scared you; we overreacted"?

When Carol and I talk with friends about the arguments in this book, they often respond with something to the effect of "What the hell? Why did the WHI investigators proceed as they did? Why did they raise frightening alarms when none were warranted? What were their motives?" And we always reply that we doubt that the investigators had nefarious goals or an intent to deceive. Rather, it seems likely that they were simply so convinced that oestrogen and HRT were harmful that they massaged their data to confirm that hypothesis. You may recall what Rowan Chlebowski, a senior WHI investigator, said when asked why the WHI had inflated the importance of breast cancer risks that were not statistically signifi-cant: He said that if it's an important question and you can't do the study again because it costs too much money, "the statistical police have to leave the room." And then there was Jacques Rossouw, who publicized his eagerness to stop the HRT bandwagon.

Steven Sloman and Philip Fernbach, in *The Knowledge Illusion: Why We Never Think Alone,* noted that "scientific attitudes are not based on rational evaluation of evidence, and therefore providing information does not change them. Attitudes are determined instead by a host of contextual and cultural factors that make them largely immune to change."[8] As I surveyed the many decades of research and debate about menopausal hormones, that is precisely what I found. Over the past seventy years, the evidence of HRT's benefits and risks—evidence converging from animal studies, human studies, observational studies, randomized controlled studies, pilot studies, and clinical studies—has pretty much remained the same. But the inter-pretations of that evidence have changed according to the "contextual and cultural factors" that, at any given time in our society, have shaped whether women and their physicians think that hormone "replace-ment" is good or bad, healthy or detrimental, feminist or antifeminist.

A different response to our argument has come from those phy-sicians, epidemiologists, and women's health activists we have written to, people whose opinions I hold in great regard, who believe that the WHI was a valuable and groundbreaking study. At their express invitation, Carol and I sent them our articles published in the *Cancer Journal* and *Climacteric* and said, "Please tell us where we are wrong. Look where we reanalyzed the WHI's own conclusions; did we go off the rails somewhere? Look at all that data mining they did to squeak out significant results. Look at how unrepresentative in age and health their sample was, yet they freely extrapolated their findings to all menopausal women. Is what they did okay with you?" Two colleagues replied, in essence, that the Women's Health Initiative was a randomized controlled study, and that's all they needed to know; whatever its flaws, it was the best research we have to date and would likely ever have. Others, taking Susan Love's position, said, in essence, "You will never persuade me that taking hormones can be beneficial for women." Most of our correspondents did not respond at all.

We understand that silence. It's a pain in the neck to explain to someone why you are committed to a hypothesis when you regard that hypothesis as being as obvious and universally accepted as the fact that the earth is round. If a flat-earther asked us to justify our position that the earth is round, we wouldn't reply, and you probably wouldn't either. Of course, serious scientists endeavor to address differences of opinion, interpretations of data, and basic hypotheses during the process of peer review and arguments in professional journals. But the more committed they are to the truths they hold to be self-evident, the less motivated they are to entertain an opponent's position. It's much easier to ignore that person's position than engage in an argument about it. And it's much easier to dismiss disconfirming evidence than accept it.

Psychologist Carole Wade, a friend and coauthor of Carol's, often used a homey example to explain scientific investigation to her college classes. "Accumulating facts to support an outdated theory in science," she said, "is like fitting a double-size sheet onto a queen-size mattress—you can get three corners to work but not the fourth. Some scientists will do everything they can to get that sheet to fit. But eventually they will need a new sheet or a new mattress." The "oestrogen causes breast cancer" evidence has become a sheet that is not fitting the bed. But if you are in the double-size-sheet business, you're going to fight like mad to get that fourth corner to work.

Cognitive psychologist Daniel Kahneman called this protective mechanism "theory-induced blindness," a condition he diagnosed in himself as well as in many of his colleagues and other scientists. "Once you have accepted a theory and used it as a tool in your thinking," he wrote, "it is extraordinarily difficult to notice its flaws. If you come upon an observation that does not seem to fit the model, you assume that there must be a perfectly good explanation that you are somehow missing. You give the theory the benefit of the doubt, trusting the community of experts who have accepted it."[9]

We are well aware that critics will accuse us of our own theory-induced blindness. Perhaps, they'll say, we are in the pocket of Big Pharma. (We are not.) Perhaps, they'll suggest, we are angry at the WHI investigators for personal reasons. (We are not.) They assume we must be biased if we are discounting the findings of the single most important study of hormone therapy, the randomized controlled trial conducted by the Women's Health Initiative.

Consumer activists and bioethicists have written extensively about the problem of conflicts of interest in research. (Carol has as well.[10]) John Ioannidis, professor of medicine and of health research and policy at Stanford University School of Medicine, has long been a powerful, eloquent voice in criticizing research in medicine that is paid for by the pharmaceutical industry, and he includes the research on HRT in that category.[11] I respect his work and I know from personal correspondence with him that he believes that the data implicating hormones as a risk of breast cancer are strong and scientifically reliable. It's certainly true that researchers who accept funding from pharmaceutical companies are more likely to get the results that their funders want, but the problem of bias in interpreting a study's results afflicts many investigators, regardless of who is paying them. In a review of 164 randomized controlled studies related to breast cancer, researchers found that "spin and bias" in interpreting results were prevalent in a high percentage of them, and the source of funding (industry or government) made no difference.[12]

In fact, the official journal of the American Society of Clinical Oncology issued a statement in 2017 underscoring the "untapped potential of observational research to inform clinical decision making," because observational studies can often answer questions that cannot or have not been answered by RCTs.[13] Thomas R. Frieden, former director of the Centers for Disease Control and Prevention, compared RCTs with other methods and identified their strengths and weaknesses. Some research methods, he wrote, are superior to RCTs and provide "valid evidence for clinical and public health action.... Elevating RCTs at the expense of other potentially highly valuable sources of data is counterproductive."[14]

That is why in this book we have drawn from a wide variety of studies to see the picture that emerges from the mosaic they create. Roger Lobo, professor of obstetrics and gynecology at the Columbia College of Physicians and Surgeons, showed that the 20 to 40 percent reduction in mortality rates for women on HRT is consistent across all scientific methods: observational meta-analyses, RCTs, the WHI itself, a Cochrane meta-analysis of randomized trials, and observational studies.[15]

The lesson is not that all research is hopelessly tainted. It is that all humans are biased—sometimes by money, sometimes by personal convictions—and that we must all do our best to critically evaluate the best scientific and clinical information that we can get.

And now, one more time, the Women's Health Initiative.

TEN KEY PROBLEMS WITH THE WOMEN'S HEALTH INITIATIVE

The U.S. Preventive Services Task Force, which creates guidelines for primary-care physicians, continues to reiterate its opposition to hormone therapy for postmenopausal women who do not have bothersome symptoms. (The USPSTP is not in fact a government-sponsored group; it consists of 16 volunteer physicians from various medical specialties. They do not conduct research; they review available evidence.) They specified that they were not going to address the use of hormones for preventing or treating menopausal symptoms; instead, their focus was to adamantly advise against the use of hormones for the prevention of chronic conditions in post-menopausal women.[16] They conceded that women taking oestrogen alone had significantly lower risks of breast cancer, diabetes, and osteoporotic fractures than women taking placebo, but these benefits, they said, were outweighed by the significantly higher risks of gallbladder disease, stroke, urinary incontinence, and venous blood clots. The task force's conclusions were based almost entirely on the findings of the Women's Health Initiative.

Because so many physicians still rely on the task force's guidelines, I want to summarize ten problems with the Women's Health Initiative that challenge its claim to gold-standard science and the validity of its conclusions:

1. The WHI rushed into publication without most of the co-investigators having seen, let alone approved, the final paper that was submitted to *JAMA*. It was fifteen years before one of those investigators published his blistering account of the violations of the scientific process and publication that the WHI and *JAMA* committed.

2. The WHI's finding that HRT increased the risk of breast cancer—the principal reason the study was halted prematurely—was not statistically significant. Yet a few of the WHI's primary investigators decided that breast cancer was such a worry for American women that it would be all right to "lower the bar" of statistical convention in this case. Press releases trumpeting the statistically nonsignificant increase in breast cancer preceded the distribution of the journal, and that scare made its way around the world before professionals could examine the evidence.

3. The study's sample was not representative of menopausal women; their average age was 63. Yet the researchers had no qualms about generalizing their conclusions and

recommendations to women entering menopause in their early fifties.

4. The study's sample was not representative of healthy women. Nearly half were current or past smokers; more than a third had been treated for high blood pressure; fully 70 percent were seriously overweight or obese.

5. The study's findings were often inconsistent and contradictory. During the first 2 years of the study, women randomized to HRT had a lower risk of breast cancer than those randomized to placebo. In 2002, the investigators reported a slight, nonsignificant increased risk of breast cancer, but only among women on HRT. In 2003, that risk was marginally significant; in 2006, that risk disappeared. Women taking only oestrogen had no increased risk at first; three years later, being on oestrogen was associated with a *lower* risk of breast cancer.

6. Some of the WHI's claims were found only by data mining, a statistical practice that is widely held to be unacceptable in scientific analysis. Data mining means that if you get a finding you aren't satisfied with, you go back into the numbers and manipulate them until you get a finding you do like.

7. The WHI claimed that oestrogen didn't even help alleviate menopausal symptoms, but given that they were not studying women in their fifties who were actually having menopausal symptoms, this conclusion was both meaningless and silly.

8. The WHI claimed that HRT increased the risk of heart problems, but that risk occurred only during the first year

of treatment and only among women who were more than 20 years postmenopause. Several years later, they revised their position and concluded that women who started HRT in the first 10 years following their last menstrual period in fact reduced their risk of coronary artery disease.

9. In 2004, the WHI raised the alarm that oestrogen increased the risk of strokes. This concern did not come at the recommendation of the WHI's own data safety and monitoring board; it was generated by the same small group that had sounded the false alarm about breast cancer. Moreover, the WHI used an extremely broad definition of *stroke;* it included transient, subtle deficits that went away in a day or two with no aftermath. When an independent reanalysis controlled for the statistical manipulations that had appeared to indicate danger, the supposed increased risk of stroke vanished.

10. Many of the WHI investigators have continued to promote alternatives to HRT that they incorrectly maintain are just as effective in preventing certain conditions: bisphosphonates and calcium for osteoporosis, statins for heart disease, physical and mental workouts for Alzheimer's, and the familiar panacea, a "healthy diet" and exercise. But as we've seen, bisphosphonates and statins have their own side effects and are not as effective in the long term as hormones. The other suggestions are no better than placebos.

For these reasons and many others, the North American Menopause Society issued a position statement noting that "hormone therapy does not need to be routinely discontinued in women aged older than 60 or 65 years and can be considered for continuation beyond age 65 years for persistent vasomotor symptoms, quality of life issues, or prevention of osteoporosis after appropriate evaluation and counseling of benefits and risks.... There are no data to support routine discontinuation in women age 65 years."[17] This position statement has been endorsed by 31 international menopause and women's health organizations, among them:

Academy of Women's Health

American Association of Clinical Endocrinologists

American Association of Nurse Practitioners

American Medical Women's Association

American Society for Reproductive Medicine

Asociación Mexicana para el Estudio del Climaterio

Association of Reproductive Health Professionals

Australasian Menopause Society

British Menopause Society

Canadian Menopause Society

Chinese Menopause Society

Colegio Mexicano de Especialistas en Ginecologia y Obstetricia

Czech Menopause and Andropause Society

Dominican Menopause Society

European Menopause and Andropause Society

German Menopause Society

Groupe d'études de la ménopause et du vieillissement hormonal

Indian Menopause Society

International Menopause Society

International Osteoporosis Foundation
International Society for the Study of Women's Sexual Health
Israeli Menopause Society
Japan Society of Menopause and Women's Health
Korean Society of Menopause
Menopause Research Society of Singapore
National Association of Nurse Practitioners in Women's
    Health
Società Italiana della Menopausa
Society of Obstetricians and Gynaecologists of Canada
South African Menopause Society
Taiwanese Menopause Society
Thai Menopause Society

The North American Menopause Society's statement advises clinicians to move away from the simplistic advice of "lowest dose for shortest time" and instead prescribe the dose and formulation based on the woman's age, time of menopause, and any unique health risks she might have. The NAMS agreed that there should be no stop date or mandatory limit on how long a woman can take HRT, and the Endocrine Society published a position paper making the same statement.[18]

I can't underscore this point strongly enough: For some conditions — notably osteoporosis and, most likely, cognitive decline — HRT's benefits stop when a woman stops taking it. A woman who had been in my breast cancer study told me that after she'd been on HRT for ten years, her doctor suggested she go off it; there was no evidence, the doctor said, of any additional benefit. But that doctor was wrong. As we saw in chapter 5, when older women stop hormones, bone loss accelerates rapidly; after six years, they have the same degree of bone loss as women who have never taken hormones.

REFLECTIONS AND RECOMMENDATIONS

Over the years, women have asked me many questions in my medical practice and in response to reading the first edition of this book. Here are a few that come up frequently.

I didn't take hormones when I entered menopause. Can I start HRT in my sixties? At the age of 64, a friend who had never taken HRT called me. "Av," she said, "I've been listening to you talk about HRT for a long time, and I'd like to go on it. It's been six years since I entered menopause, and I've had no symptoms, but I'm concerned about my memory, my heart, and my sex life. Should I consider starting it now?"

It's a logical question. My position is that women who begin HRT during menopause for symptoms that seriously affect the quality of their lives have no reason not to take it for as long as it's beneficial and for as many years as they wish — under the guidance of their physicians, of course. But HRT isn't something a woman should start and stop every few years. It's not candy or a vitamin. There is a window of opportunity, roughly defined as the first ten years after a woman's last menstrual period, during which HRT has its greatest benefits. There may be an elevated risk for women who begin taking it more than ten years after menopause; if they have any preexisting atherosclerotic plaques, there is a risk of further obstructing an already narrowed artery, at least during the first year of HRT. This risk can be assessed with tests that determine arterial health and heart strength. I therefore encouraged my friend to have the tests; she passed with flying colors and began HRT. But I would not have been comfortable advising her to take hormones without that precaution.

What about the risks of HRT? Yes, there are risks. Most are minor, such as dry eyes (curiously, also a symptom of menopause).[19] Some women suffer migraine headaches during menstruation, and taking oestrogen can lead to a return of those headaches.[20] Some risks are more serious; as the U.S. Preventive Services Task Force noted, they include gallbladder disease and venous blood clots. But as Roger Lobo summarized, "Many of the adverse effects are not life-threatening and can be dealt with by adjusting the dose and preparation of HRT. These effects include breast tenderness, abdominal bloating, mood changes, uterine bleeding and an idiosyncratic elevation in blood pressure that might occur with oral oestrogens." He noted that more serious concerns such as venous thromboembolism (a blood clot in a vein that migrates to the lungs) might occur, but in healthy women entering menopause, "these risks are small or not significantly increased over placebo treatment.... The available data suggest no increased risks or serious adverse effects of HRT."[21]

In 2021, the WHI reported finding no difference between women on hormones (oestrogen alone or HRT) and those on placebo in their risk of venous clots or pulmonary embolism.[22] A growing number of professional organizations endorse Lobo's conclusions, regarding risks as being dwarfed by HRT's benefits for heart, bones, brain, and longevity. The British Menopause Society and Women's Health Concern recommended that arbitrary limits should not be placed on how long women used HRT. If symptoms persisted, their statement noted, "the benefits of hormone therapy usually outweigh the risks."[23]

Aren't there other good ways of treating the symptoms of menopause? In chapter 1 we noted that menopausal symptoms may affect up to 80 percent of perimenopausal and postmenopausal women and that these symptoms last an average of seven years, longer for Black women. While most symptoms eventually clear with time, the symptoms associated with urogenital atrophy, including vaginal itching, urinary burning, urinary frequency, and painful sexual intercourse, become more pronounced as a woman grows older. These symptoms can often be treated successfully with topical oestrogen creams. Herbal remedies benefit about 20 percent of women — the same success rate as placebo. Neurontin, an anti-seizure medication, and Paxil, an antidepressant, reduce hot flushes in about 60 percent of women, but they do not help other menopausal symptoms, such as joint pains, insomnia, and heart palpitations.

Can't I just take the lowest dose for the shortest time? There is no scientific basis for this recommendation, although it still appears on all preparations of oestrogen.

How should I think about my symptoms and decide if HRT is right for me? If you are in perimenopause or menopause and considering HRT as a way to improve your quality of life, begin by reviewing the symptoms listed at the start of chapter 1. Be sure to take note not only of familiar symptoms like hot flushes and night sweats but also those symptoms not usually associated with menopause, such as joint pain, heart palpitations, headaches, depression, and insomnia. Ask yourself: "How severe is each symptom? How much does that symptom affect my quality of life — not at all, it's tolerable, it's pretty bad, or it's unbearable?" Next, consider other factors that might influence your decision, such as whether your mother suffered from osteoporosis, heart disease, or cognitive decline.

Why not take statins instead of HRT to protect my heart? As we discussed in chapter 4, heart disease is the leading killer of women in every decade of life after age 40. Heart disease is responsible for more deaths than breast cancer—even among breast cancer survivors. Being on oestrogen or HRT can reduce the risk of cardiovascular events and death by up to 50 percent. Most medical organizations counsel against using hormones to protect heart health, instead advising statins to reduce cholesterol and anti-arrhythmia drugs to control palpitations. But statins do not reduce a woman's risk of having a *first* heart attack, and these drugs are not free from potentially serious side effects. Statins may cause diabetes or liver damage, and anti-arrhythmics may cause unacceptable slowing of the heart rate.

Why not take calcium and bisphosphonates to prevent osteoporosis and bone fractures? The number of female deaths annually in the United States associated with osteoporotic hip fractures is approximately the same as the number of deaths from breast cancer. As we saw in chapter 5, oestrogen reduces the risk of osteoporotic hip fractures by 30 to 50 percent, but women should remain on hormones for at least ten years to achieve this benefit; according to some experts, they should continue hormones indefinitely. While calcium and vitamin D may be helpful to avoid hip fractures in premenopausal women who also exercise, they are of no appreciable benefit for postmenopausal women who are not taking HRT. There is no association between calcium, vitamin D, or combined calcium and vitamin D supplements and the incidence of nonvertebral, vertebral, or total fractures. Bisphosphonates, whether taken by mouth or by injection, do decrease the risk of hip fractures at first, but, paradoxically, they increase the fracture risk after five years. In addition, they can cause stomach upset and, rarely, a serious and painful loss of bone in the jaw region. Evista (raloxifene) has been approved for the prevention of osteoporosis, but unlike oestrogen, it has not been shown to affect the risk of hip fractures.

What about taking estradiol and other bioidenticals instead of Premarin? I am not comfortable with the whole "mares' urine" business. We addressed this widespread concern in chapter 1, but it bears repeating. *Bioidentical* refers to prescription hormones that have the same molecular structure as hormones that are naturally produced by the body. Adult women produce estradiol, the most prominent circulating oestrogen, along with estriol and estrone. (*Bioidentical oestrogen* usually refers to estradiol but it can also refer to estriol or estrone.) Premarin, the most commonly marketed form of oestrogen, is extracted from pregnant mares' urine, a source that makes some women uncomfortable; however, it contains at least ten molecular forms of oestrogen. Roberta Diaz Brinton and her colleagues have long been studying oestrogen and brain function in relation to Alzheimer's, and they discovered that equilin, a form of oestrogen that is found only in Premarin, stimulates the growth of neurons in the cortex and other regions of the brain.[24]

Commercially manufactured oestrogen and bioidentical oestrogen (usually estradiol) are both approved and regulated by the FDA. In contrast, *compounded* bioidentical hormones, which are widely used in the United States, are generally prepared by local pharmacies in response to a prescription written by a woman's physician. They are not standardized pharmaceutical products and are not regulated by the FDA. That is why I, along with all major medical societies, discourage their use as an alternative to approved forms of oestrogen and progesterone.

Does the form of oestrogen that I take make a difference? Many women who are on HRT are taking oestrogen in the form of a patch rather than as a pill, and they often ask me if that is okay. The reason they take oestrogen in this form is usually that their gynecologists tell them that the patch is not as harmful because it doesn't increase the risk of clots. That is true, but what they don't add is that the patch is not as helpful either. Not all forms of oestrogen have equal benefits on cognitive function, for example, or on reducing heart disease. The oral form appears to be mildly more beneficial than the patch in preventing cardiovascular disease and stroke.[25] In 2021, the WHI reported finding no difference between women on hormones (oestrogen alone or HRT) and those on placebo in their risk of venous clots or pulmonary embolism.[26]

What about exercise, mental and physical, to reduce my risk of dementia and cognitive decline? Whereas deaths from heart disease, strokes, and breast cancer are falling, the number of deaths associated with Alzheimer's disease is steadily rising, especially among women. As we saw in chapter 6, no nonhormonal treatment is effective in slowing or reversing the tragic symptoms of Alzheimer's and other dementias—not drugs, not mental exercises, not even physical workouts. The only promising intervention at present is oestrogen, if it is begun during the "menopause window" and continued for at least ten years.

Is progesterone a problem? For many years, it was the use of oestrogen that was believed to put postmenopausal women at increased risk of developing breast cancer. Now we are learning that that isn't so; oestrogen might even decrease that risk. So attention turned to the possible harms of progesterone. When women take oestrogen combined with micronized progesterone, no increased risk of breast cancer has thus far been observed in any study. While I don't agree with them, some investigators believe there is a very small increased risk when the form of progesterone is synthetic progestin, but even so, it is no more than 2 percent. And even if HRT increases the risk of breast cancer by this modest increment, recall that women on HRT live, on average, years longer than those not taking HRT.

What are the benefits and risks of testosterone for reducing meno-pausal symptoms and increasing sexual desire? In 2016, psychologists at Emory University reported that oestrogen therapy, which achieves premenopausal levels of oestrogen, increases sexual desire in postmenopausal women. Testosterone given in doses achieving higher than normal levels enhances the effectiveness of oestrogen in stimulating sexual desire.[27] However, the International Society for the Study of Women's Sexual Health cautioned that although "current available research supports a moderate therapeutic bene-fit" for testosterone, "long-term safety has not been established."[28] And what is a "moderate therapeutic benefit"? A review of random-ized clinical trials found that the therapeutic use of testosterone for low sexual desire in women resulted in approximately one addi-tional satisfactory sexual activity per month, and "there is currently insufficient evidence regarding general recommendations for tes-tosterone therapy in women."[29]

Given that insufficient evidence, it is no wonder that findings are conflicting, particularly on the question of breast cancer. Some studies suggest that elevated circulating levels of testosterone raises the risk of a new breast cancer or its recurrence,[30] but these reports have not been consistent. Other studies, including a literature review from the London Breast Institute and those by Rebecca Glaser at Wright State University, suggest that testosterone may reduce the risk of breast cancer.[31]

I wish I had scientifically validated answers for the risks and benefits of testosterone, but I don't, nor do I trust those who claim they do. That is why I advise caution for women thinking of taking testosterone and for physicians eager to prescribe it.

I've had breast cancer but I'm now in menopause and having some terrible symptoms. Can I safely take HRT? Yes. (Read chapter 3, then talk to your doctor.)

The Process of Science and the Art of Medicine

Sir George White Pickering, a British medical doctor and professor of medicine at the University of Oxford, understood well the conflicting demands on every physician who seeks to help patients with the best available scientific information. "If you are a clinician," he said, "you must believe that you know what will help your patient; otherwise, you cannot counsel, you cannot prescribe. If you are a scientist, however, you must be uncertain—a scientist who no longer asks questions is a bad scientist."[32]

For me, the practice of medicine is like walking a tightrope, balancing between art and science, certainty and uncertainty; here's a drug or regimen that benefits patients overall, but some individuals will not do well on it. For any treatment, we physicians are always calculating whether the benefits outweigh the risks and wondering how that calculation might be customized for any given patient. Science, after all, gives us overall patterns and predictions for groups; it can't tell us what a particular individual should do. That's why smokers are forever pointing to their aunt Sally or great-uncle Morty who smoked three packs a day and lived to be 99; they rely on the outlying exception to justify smoking and ignore the more important statistic, namely the immense risk to their own health. Conversely, some women say, "My friend Harriet took HRT for five years and got breast cancer, so I'll never consider it." They are relying on an understandably compelling anecdote, but one that doesn't conform to the greater evidence. And if Harriet hadn't taken HRT, can we be sure she would not have gotten breast cancer? And if Harriet had drunk coffee every morning for five years and then got breast cancer, would that be a reason to forgo coffee?

I draw insight from the kitten study, which is rather like the neurological counterpart of Kahneman's notion of theory-induced blindness. Like human infants, kittens are born with the visual ability to detect horizontal and vertical lines and other spatial orientations. But if they are deprived of normal visual experience, these cells deteriorate and the cats' perception suffers. In one classic study, kittens were reared in darkness for five months after birth, but for several hours each day, they were put into a special cylinder that permitted them to see only vertical or horizontal lines. Later, the cats that had been exposed only to horizontal lines had trouble perceiving vertical ones; they would run to play with horizontal bars but not vertical bars.[33] Give them a chair, and they would jump onto its horizontal seat but repeatedly bump into its legs. Give the "vertical" kittens the same chair, and they would happily weave around its legs but literally not see the horizontal seat to curl up on.

I have often observed how mental blinders can prevent physicians and patients from seeing the whole picture. I understand why many people are distrustful of modern medicine, which often seems a coldhearted enterprise involving technology and medications administered by busy physicians who lack the time to focus on the human beings in front of them—the human beings who are full of uncertainty, worry, and fear. I understand why so many people today are drawn to alternative medicine, with its promises of "natural" remedies, "bioidentical" compounds, and humanistic concerns for the whole person. But just as a healthy kitten needs to perceive the legs *and* the seat of that chair, a single perception on its own distorts one's field of vision.

I see my patients as being far more than the immediate problem they come in with; I temper what I've learned from science with what I've learned about human beings. Like all oncologists, I am fully aware of the toll that breast cancer exacts on women, their loved ones, and the general population. But I do not want that concern to dominate my advice or plan of treatment for any given woman. Some HRT researchers and breast cancer activists are like the vertical-line kittens, able to focus only on breast cancer and their patients' fear of breast cancer; breast cancer is *all* they fear and all they see. But this focus can lead to a failure to consider women's greater risk of suffering from heart disease and osteoporosis, conditions that are far more likely to be fatal. A diagnosis of breast cancer is no longer inevitably a death sentence, and it hasn't been for decades. Successful treatment most often no longer requires a mastectomy; the majority of patients are now treated without chemotherapy; and, as I keep repeating, more than 90 percent of women diagnosed with early breast cancer today are likely to be cured. A woman's life situation, symptoms, risk of other illnesses, and personal goals must be factored into any recommendations for taking oestrogen, as should the form, dose, and duration of that treatment.

For that reason, I would never presume to advise readers of a book—even this one—of their best or healthiest course of action. Nevertheless, as someone who has spent his life walking that tightrope between science and practice, I am convinced of the immense benefits of HRT, including its likely ability to prolong women's lives. For women's health and quality of life, for better science and medical practice, it's time to retire outdated beliefs about oestrogen. Women should not be taking HRT because of Robert Wilson's impossible and patronizing notion that it will make them "feminine forever." But, as Bernadine Healy advised so many years ago, it is likely to make them healthier longer. That's why there's no question in my mind that oestrogen matters.

Epilogue

Martha, Medicine, and Making Decisions

This book began with my story about my wife's breast cancer and our mutual decision, made three years after she finished treatment, that she would begin HRT. People often ask me, "What happened with Martha? How is she?," and I feel I owe them, and you, the full story.

Martha's chemotherapy, more than thirty-five years ago, pushed her into early menopause, which came with many of its familiar symptoms, including hot flushes, insomnia, palpitations, and cognitive deficits. She was resigned to most of them but she found the cognitive problems, notably trouble reading and remembering, intolerable. Three years posttreatment, she was strong and active, in overall good health, and, we believed, cancer-free, and so we discussed the possible risks and benefits of her beginning HRT. Though we did not have the benefit at that time of the research discussed in this book, she decided to enroll in the study I had just begun, of giving HRT to breast cancer survivors. The hormones completely reversed all her menopausal symptoms, and she stayed on HRT for 26 years.

And then Martha had a small recurrence at the site of her original breast cancer—an extremely rare phenomenon. With no evidence of spread, the tumor was removed surgically and she needed no other treatment. But now we had to decide whether she should resume HRT. I'll let Martha explain:

"There is absolutely no way to know whether three decades of HRT caused this recurrence, delayed it, or played no role at all. What I did know was that I'd had 26 years of really good health and I had not experienced the bone fractures, heart disease, and dementia that plagued my mother during the same decades of her life. Most important for me, my memory and cognition were as sharp as ever. Looking back, I would not change the decision we made when I first dealt with breast cancer years ago."

But after the recurrence, Martha and I decided she would not go back on HRT unless she felt she was having cognitive problems. Nearly six years later, she is still off hormones and I can testify that her mind and memory are indeed as sharp as ever. Was there a benefit to her overall health as a result of the long-term HRT treatment? Did HRT allow her to escape the heart, bone, and brain diseases that afflicted her mother? It feels that way, but we will never know for sure.

Martha's attitude reflects the complexity of making any decision where the outcome is not 100 percent certain, which is most of them. Every action you take involves risk: crossing the street, swallowing an aspirin, getting vaccinated, getting married. In the case of HRT, yes, there are some legitimate concerns about risks, as we have seen. But we should not extrapolate from one person's experience, good or bad, to everyone's. Too many medical professionals, concerned about what turns out to be small risks for *some* women, overlook the overwhelming evidence of oestrogen's large benefits for *most* women. We hope this book will provide readers with a deeper understanding that will allow every woman, with guidance from an informed and empathic physician, to make decisions based on knowledge and evidence rather than on unfounded anxiety and false alarms.

Acknowledgments

From Avrum:

The first person I want to thank is Carol. During the course of our long friendship, we have coauthored scientific papers, editorials, and book reviews, and, knowing the long-standing importance of this issue to me and for women's health, she set her sights on helping me write this book. It is her persistence, her insights, her merciless critical appraisals, her sense of humor, and her talent as a writer that brought this book to life.

It can be daunting to hold and espouse a minority opinion in medicine, but I never felt alone. I am grateful to the late Phil DiSaia, former president of the American Board of Obstetrics and Gynecology and professor in the School of Medicine at UC Irvine, who wrote about the benefits and risks of HRT years before I did, published one of the earliest studies of HRT administered to breast cancer survivors, and always supported my efforts in this area. Other physicians who have helped me both by example and with advice are Michael Baum, Howard Hodis, V. Craig Jordan, Matteo Lambertini, Robert Langer, Roger Lobo, Louise Newson, JoAnn Pinkerton, Serge Rozenberg, Richard Santen, Philip Sarrel, Basil

Stoll, Rena Vassilopoulou-Sellin, and Dietrich von Fournier. I also wish to thank the physicians across diverse specialties who offered encouragement and counsel, notably Peter Attia, Jonathan Berek, David Decker, Marc Espie, Faith Fitzgerald, and John Stevenson, along with colleagues and friends who read earlier versions of this argument and provided many helpful suggestions: Judy Baldwin, Peter Clarke, Susan Evans, Patricia T. Kelly, and Nancy Reaven.

I am also indebted to the physicians who have been leaders in restoring a balanced view of HRT's benefits and risks, for the public as well as their colleagues: Kelly Casperson, Alberto Dominguez-Bali, Sarah Glynne, Marie Claire Haver, Heather Hirsch, Sharon Malone, Corinne Menn, Lila Nachtigall, Rachel Rubin, Mache Seibel, James Simon, and Vonda Wright. They and I have been supported by informed and often outspoken women who have shared their experiences fighting to obtain prescriptions for HRT, including Debora Bitticks, Saundra DeCrescent, Diana Hawthorne, Mish Kaplan, Dena Kaye, Doreen Seidler-Feller, Myra Straussman, Katie Taylor, Ann Trygstad, and Sally Zamarin.

I am deeply grateful to the many members of the Los Angeles medical community, most especially those affiliated with the current Providence Cedars-Sinai Tarzana Regional Medical Center, at which I served as director of oncology, chief of staff, and director of continuing medical education. These colleagues listened patiently to my opinions and encouraged my continued study of HRT for breast cancer survivors. Among the many people who made it possible for me to swim upstream by publishing my ideas in professional journals or giving me a public forum for debate are Edward Bouwer, Ken Frazier, Phyllis Greenberger, Val Jones, Michael J. Mastrangelo, Saar Porrath, Nancy Raymon, Erik Rifkin, Selma

Schimmel, Mel Silverstein, Steven Strauss, and Michael Van Scoy-Mosher. My special thanks to Vince DeVita, editor in chief of the *Cancer Journal,* who spent Christmas Eve reading Carol's and my first paper on HRT and who called the next morning to say he had recommended it be published.

Finally, warm thanks to N. J. Nakamura, the oncology nurse-practitioner in my office who was our study coordinator, and Sarah Viscuso, research librarian at Providence.org., who provided citations and full text papers within hours of every request.

From Avrum and Carol:

We want to express our gratitude to Jane Isay, the much-admired book editor and publisher with whom Carol once worked. Over lunch in New York, listening to Carol talk about Avrum's work, Jane nearly dropped her fork. "It's a book!" she exclaimed. "A medical mystery story — *Who Killed HRT?*" That title didn't survive the conversation, but the idea did. In a heartbeat Jane introduced us to Gail Ross, now at the William Morris Endeavor Agency, who became our literary agent as soon as she learned about our project. In a world full of people grousing about their agents, we could not be more pleased by our experience working with Gail and her staff, especially Dara Kaye, who did superb editing on our initial book proposal. Gail took on our project with alacrity and has remained an enthusiastic supporter and adviser. She got us to Tracy Behar, then publisher and editor in chief of Little, Brown Spark, who introduced herself by saying, "I am your ideal reader." And she has been — and our ideal editor as well. She raised important conceptual concerns and never pressed us to sacrifice evidence for the sake of making the book more "pop medicine." As we finished this edition, she moved on to newer pastures, leaving us in the capable hands of Michael Szczerban. We have had a superb experience with everyone we have worked with: executive production editor Linda Arends, who expertly steered the manuscript through the shoals of production; editorial assistant Karina Leon, who answered every question and facilitated the process with warmth and efficiency; art director Lucy Kim, who designed the original eye-catching cover and updated it perfectly for this edition; Tracy Roe, the undisputed queen of copyediting, whose close and informed reading enhanced and clarified the text; and the meticulous work of our exceptional proofreader, Barbara Jatkola. Our thanks to the entire Little, Brown Spark team for making the experience of writing this book so gratifying and pleasurable.

Finally, our warmest thanks to Adam Bluming and Stephanie Kemp of NELA Films for the elegant design of the book's website and for producing its videos; to Ariel Margolis, the mastermind behind our social media presence and platform success; and to Kathy Jacobi, for taking the warm headshots that adorn the book jacket. It takes a village to write a book too, and we are grateful for ours.

Notes

Introduction: Who Killed HRT?

1. Goldman L, Tosteson AN. Uncertainty about postmenopausal estrogen: Time for action, not debate. N Engl J Med. 1991;325:-800–802.

2. Col NF, Eckman MH, Karas RH, et al. Patient-specific decisions about hormone replacement therapy in postmenopausal women. JAMA. 1997;277:1140–47.

3. Healy, Bernadine, *A New Prescription for Women's Health: Getting the Best Medical Care in a Man's World* (New York: Viking, 1995), 200–201.

4. Rossouw JE, Anderson GL, Prentice RL, et al. Risks and benefits of estrogen plus progestin in healthy postmenopausal women: Principal results from the Women's Health Initiative Randomized Controlled Trial. JAMA. 2002;288:321–33.

5. Ettinger B, Wang SM, Leslie RS, et al. Evolution of postmenopausal hormone therapy between 2002 and 2009. Menopause. 2012;19:610–15.

6. Brown S. Shock, terror and controversy: How the media reacted to the Women's Health Initiative. Climacteric. 2012;15:275–80.

7. Hays J, Ockene JK, Brunner RL, et al. for the Women's Health Initiative Investigators. Effect of estrogen plus progestin on health-related quality of life. N Engl J Med. 2003;348:1839–54.

8. Bluming AZ, Tavris C. Hormone replacement therapy: Real concerns and false alarms. Cancer J. 2009;15:93–104.

   Bluming AZ, Tavris C. What are the real risks for breast cancer? Climacteric. 2012;15:133–38.

   Bluming AZ, Tavris C. Chains of evidence, mosaics of data: Does estrogen *cause* breast cancer? How would we know? Climacteric. 2012;15:531–37.

9. In 2005, a lawyer representing Wyeth contacted Avrum and asked him to be an expert witness on a case; Avrum agreed, since his already published papers had questioned the role of hormones in the development of breast cancer. He was not hired to create an opinion.

10. Shifren JL, Crandall CJ, Manson JE. Menopausal hormone therapy. JAMA. 2019;321:2458–59.

11. Stuenkel CA, Manson JE. Women's Health—Traversing medicine and public policy. N Engl J Med. 2021;384:2073–76.

   Flores VA, Pal L, Manson JE. Hormone Therapy in Menopause: Concepts, Controversies, and Approach to Treatment. Endocr Rev. 2021 Nov 16;42(6):720–52.

12. Chlebowski RT, Anderson GL, Aragaki AK. Association of menopausal hormone therapy with breast cancer incidence and mortality during long-term follow-up of the Women's Health Initiative Randomized Clinical Trials. JAMA. 2020;324:369–80.

13. Hodis HN, Sarrel PM. Menopausal hormone therapy and breast cancer: What is the evidence from randomized trials? Climacteric. 2018;21:521–28.

   Bluming AZ, Hodis HN, Langer RD. 'Tis but a scratch: A critical review of the WHI evidence associating menopausal hormone therapy with the risk of breast cancer. Menopause. 2023; 30(12):183–90.

NOTES

Chapter 1: The "Change of Life" and the Quality of Life

1. *O, The Oprah Magazine,* August 2002; http://www.oprah.com /omagazine/be-aware-for-perimenopause/all.
2. Loh, Sandra Tsing, *The Madwoman in the Volvo* (New York: W. W. Norton, 2014), 15.
3. Parker-Pope, Tara, *The Hormone Decision* (Emmaus, PA: Rodale, 2007), 133.
4. Utian WH, Gass ML, Pickar JH. Body mass index does not influence response to treatment, nor does body weight change with lower doses of conjugated estrogens and medroxyprogesterone acetate in early postmenopausal women. Menopause. 2004;11:306–14.

    Barnabei VM, Cochrane BB, Aragaki AK, et al. Menopausal symptoms and treatment-related effects of estrogen and progestin in the Women's Health Initiative. Obstet Gynecol. 2005;105:1063–73.
5. Watkins, Elizabeth S., *The Estrogen Elixir: A History of Hormone Replacement Therapy in America* (Baltimore: Johns Hopkins University Press, 2007), 1.
6. Marriott LK, Wenk GL. Neurobiological consequences of long-term estrogen therapy. Curr Dir Psychol Sci. 2004;13:173–76.
7. Watkins, *The Estrogen Elixir,* 185.
8. Ibid.
9. Kolata, Gina, "Hormone Therapy, Already Found to Have Risks, Is Now Said to Lack Benefits," *New York Times,* March 18, 2003.
10. Nachtigall L. Treatment of estrogen deficiency symptoms in women surviving breast cancer. Part 4. Urogenital atrophy, vasomotor instability, sleep disorders, and related symptoms. Oncol. 1999;13:551–75.
11. Grob, Gerald N. and Horwitz, Allan V., *Diagnosis, Therapy, and Evidence: Conundrums in Modern American Medicine* (New Brunswick, NJ: Rutgers University Press, 2010), 195.
12. Wilson, Robert A., *Feminine Forever* (New York: Pocket Books, 1966).

13. Kolata, Gina, with Petersen, Melody, "Hormone Replacement Study a Shock to the Medical System," *New York Times,* July 10, 2002.

14. Martin, Emily, *The Woman in the Body: A Cultural Analysis of Reproduction* (Boston: Beacon, 1987).

15. Mosconi, Lisa, *The Menopause Brain* (New York: Avery, 2024).

16. Wood BM, et al. Demographic and hormonal evidence for menopause in wild chimpanzees. Science. 2023;382:368–69.

17. Hrdy, Sarah Blaffer, *Mother Nature: Maternal Instincts and How They Shape the Human Species* (New York: Ballantine, 1999).

18. Avis NE, Crawford SL, Greendale G, et al. Duration of menopausal vasomotor symptoms over the menopause transition. JAMA Intern Med. 2015;175:531–39.

19. Gupta, Alisha, "Menopause Is Different for Women of Color," *New York Times,* August 23, 2023.

20. Hays J, Ockene JK, Brunner RL, et al. Effects of estrogen plus progestin on health-related quality of life. N Engl J Med. 2003;348:1839–54.

21. Ibid., 1839.

22. Watkins, *The Estrogen Elixir,* 1.

23. Nelson HD. Commonly used types of postmenopausal estrogen for treatment of hot flashes: Scientific review. JAMA. 2004;291:1610–20.

24. Welton AJ, Vickers MR, Kim J, et al. Health-related quality of life after combined hormone replacement therapy: Randomized controlled trial. BMJ. 2008;337:a1190.

25. Ockene JK, Barad DH, Cochrane BB, et al. Symptom experience after discontinuing use of estrogen plus progestin. JAMA. 2005;294:183–93.

26. Christgau S, Tanko LB, Cloos PA, et al. Suppression of elevated cartilage turnover in postmenopausal women and in ovariectomized rats by estrogen and a selective estrogen-receptor modulator (SERM). Menopause. 2004;11:508–18.

27. Schmidt PJ, Nieman L, Danaceau MA, et al. Estrogen replacement in perimenopause-related depression: A preliminary report. Am J Obstet Gynecol. 2000;183:414–20.

Soares CN, Almeida OP, Joffe H, et al. Efficacy of estradiol for the treatment of depressive disorders in perimenopausal women: a double-blind, randomized, placebo-controlled trial. Arch Gen Psychiatry. 2001;58:529–34.

28. Kirsch I. Antidepressants and the placebo effect. Z Psychol [in English]. 2014;222:128–34.

29. Taylor, Katie, "Finding the Positive Side of Menopause," *Jewish Chronicle*, May 12, 2007; https://www.pressreader.com/uk/the-jewish-chronicle/20170512/282127816396074.

30. ACOG Practice Bulletin No. 141: Management of menopausal symptoms. Obstet Gynecol. 2014;123:202–16.

31. The 2017 hormone therapy position statement of the North American Menopause Society. Menopause. 2017;24:728–53.

32. Langer RD, Manson JE, Allison MA. Have we come full circle—or moved forward? The Women's Health Initiative 10 years on. Climacteric. 2012;15:206–12.

Utian WH. A decade post WHI, menopausal hormone therapy comes full circle—need for independent commission. Climacteric. 2012;15:320–25.

33. Smyth, Chris, "Women Told Hormone Replacement Therapy Does Not Lead to Early Death," *Times* (UK), September 13, 2017.

34. Richard-Davis G, Manson JE. Vasomotor symptom duration in midlife women—research overturns dogma. JAMA Intern Med. 2015;175:540–41.

35. Flores VA, Pal L, Manson JE. Hormone Therapy in Menopause: Concepts, Controversies, and Approach to Treatment. Endocr Rev. 2021;42(6):720–52; https://doi.org/10.1210/endrev/bnab-011doi.

36. Crandall CJ, Mehta JM, Manson JE. Management of menopausal symptoms. A Review. JAMA. 2023;329:405–20.

37. Grand View Research, "Menopause Market Size, Share and Trends Analysis Report by Treatment"; https://www.grandviewresearch.com/industry-analysis/menopause-market.

38. Santen RJ, Stuenkel CA, Davis SR, et al. Managing menopausal symptoms and associated clinical issues in breast cancer survivors. J Clin Endocrinol Metab. 2017;102:3647–61; https://doi.org/10.1210/jc.2017-01138.

39. Pollack A. "F.D.A. Panel Advises Against Two Medicines to Treat Hot Flashes," *New York Times,* March 4, 2013. See also "Gabapentin for Hot Flashes," *Medical News Today,* April 2022; https://www.medicalnewstoday.com/articles/gabapentin-for-hot-flashes.

40. Carroll DG, Kelley KW. Use of antidepressants for management of hot flashes. Pharmacotherapy. 2009;29:1357–74.

41. Quinlan, Ailin, "The Menopause—Everything You Need to Know about the Change," *Irish Independent,* June 19, 2017.

42. Tice JA, Ettinger B, Ensrud K, et al. Phytoestrogen supplements for the treatment of hot flashes: The Isoflavone Clover Extract Study: A randomized controlled trial. JAMA. 2003;290:207–14.

43. Grady D. Management of menopausal symptoms. N Engl J Med. 2006;355:2338–47.

44. Nelson HD, Vesco KK, Haney E, et al. Nonhormonal therapies for menopausal hot flashes: Systematic review and meta-analysis. JAMA. 2006;295:2057–71.

45. Newton KM, Reed SD, LaCroix AZ, et al. Treatment of vasomotor symptoms of menopause with black cohosh, multi-botanicals, soy, hormone therapy, or placebo. Ann Int Med. 2006;145:869–79.

   Mangione C. A randomized trial of alternative medicines for vasomotor symptoms of menopause. Ann Int Med. 2006;145:924–25.

46. Pockaj BA, Gallagher JG, Loprinzi CL, et al. Phase III double-blind, randomized, placebo-controlled crossover trial of black cohosh in the management of hot flashes: NCCTG trial N01CC. J Clin Oncol. 2006;18:2836–41.

47. Herbal medicines for menopausal symptoms. Drug Ther Bull. 2009;47:2–6.
48. Schwartz, Erika, Holtorf, Kent, and Brownstein, David, "The Truth about Hormone Therapy," *Wall Street Journal,* March 16, 2009.
49. Brinton RD, Proffitt P, Tran J, et al. Equilin, a principal component of the estrogen replacement therapy Premarin, increases the growth of cortical neurons via an NMDA receptor-dependent mechanism. Exp Neurol. 1997;147:211–20.
50. Santoro N, Braunstein GD, Butts CL. Compounded bioidentical hormones in endocrinology practice: An Endocrine Society scientific statement. J Clin Endocrinol Metab. 2016;101:1318–43.
51. For the full report, see National Academies of Sciences, Engineering, and Medicine 2020. The Clinical Utility of Compounded Bioidentical Hormone Therapy: A Review of Safety, Effectiveness, and Use. Washington, DC: National Academies Press.
    Stuenkel CA, Manson JE. Compounded bioidentical hormone therapy: The National Academies weigh in. JAMA Internal Medicine. December 14, 2020;7232. doi.org/10.17226/25791.
52. Ramin, Catherine J., "The hormone hoax thousands fall for." *More.com,* October 2013, 134–144, 156.
53. Thompson JJ, Ritenbaugh C, Richter M. Why women choose compounded bioidentical hormone therapy: Lessons from a qualitative study of menopause decision-making. BMC Women's Health. 2017;17:97.
54. Rosenthal MS. The Wiley Protocol: An analysis of ethical issues. Menopause. 2008;15:1014–22.
55. Hill, Amelia, "Female Doctors in Menopause Retiring Early Due to Sexism, Study Says," *The Guardian*, August 5, 2020.
56. Otterman, Sharon, "A Movement to Make Workplaces 'Menopause Friendly,'" *New York Times,* May 22, 2023.
57. Faubion, SS, Shufelt C. The menopause management vacuum. Cancer J. 2022;28:191–95.
58. Quoted in Smyth, "Women Told Hormone Replacement Therapy."

Chapter 2: Does Oestrogen Cause Breast Cancer?

1. Bluming AZ. Treatment of primary breast cancer without mastectomy. Review of the Literature. Amer J Med. 1982;72:820–28.
2. Lavecchia C, Negri E, Bruzzi P, et al. The role of age at menarche and at menopause on breast cancer risk. Combined evidence from four case-control studies. Ann Oncol. 1992;3:625–29.
3. Gail MH, Benichou J. Assessing the risk of breast cancer in individuals. Cancer Prev. 1991;1:1–15.
4. MacMahon B, Cole P, Lin M, et al. Age at first birth and breast cancer risk. Bull WHO. 1970;43:209–21.
5. Lambertini M, Kroman N, Ameye L, et al. Long-term safety of pregnancy following breast cancer according to estrogen receptor status. J Natl Cancer Inst. 2018;110:426–29.
6. Lambertini M, Ameye L, Hamy AS, et al. Pregnancy after breast cancer in patients with germline BRCA mutations. J Clin Oncol. 2020;38:3012–23.
7. King RM, Welch JS, Martin JK Jr., et al. Carcinoma of the breast associated with pregnancy. Surg Gynecol Obstet. 1985;160:228–32.
8. Partridge AH, et al. Interrupting endocrine therapy to attempt pregnancy after breast cancer. N Engl J Med. 2023;388:1645–56.
9. Clarke RB, Howell A, Potten CS, Anderson E. Dissociation between steroid receptor expression and cell proliferation in the human breast. Cancer Res. 1997;57:4987–91.

   Sleeman KE, Kendrick H, Robertson D, et al. Dissociation of estrogen receptor expression and in vivo stem cell activity in the mammary gland. J Cell Biol. 2007;176:19–26.
10. Feynman, Richard P., *The Meaning of It All: Thoughts of a Citizen Scientist* (Reading, MA: Perseus, 1998), 71.
11. Love RR, Philips J. Oophorectomy for breast cancer: History revisited. J Natl Cancer Inst. 2002;94:1433–34.

12. Smith DC, Prentice R, Thompson DJ, et al. Association of exogenous estrogen and endometrial carcinoma. N Engl J Med. 1975;293:1164–67.
13. Gambrell RD. Prevention of endometrial cancer with progestogens. Maturitas. 1986;8:159–68.
14. Brinton LA, Hoover R, and Fraumeni JF. Menopausal oestrogens and breast cancer risk: An expanded case-control study. Br J Cancer. 1986;54:825–32.
15. Armstrong BK. Estrogen therapy after the menopause: Boon or bane? Med J Aust. 1988;148:213–14.
16. Palmer JR, Rosenberg L, Clark EA, et al. Breast cancer risk after estrogen replacement therapy: Results from the Toronto breast cancer study. Am J Epidemiol. 1991;134:1386–95.
17. Dupont WD, Page DL. Menopausal estrogen replacement therapy and breast cancer. Arch Intern Med. 1991;151:67–72.
18. Nachtigall MJ, Smilen SW, Nachtigall RD, et al. Incidence of breast cancer in a 22-year study of women receiving estrogen-progestin replacement therapy. Obstet Gynecol. 1992;80:827–30.
19. Stanford JL, Weiss NS, Voight LF, et al. Combined estrogen and progestin hormone replacement therapy in relation to risk of breast cancer in middle-aged women. JAMA. 1995;274:137–42.
20. Colditz GA, Hankinson SE, Hunter DJ, et al. The use of estrogens and progestins and the risk of breast cancer in postmenopausal women. N Engl J Med. 1995;332:1589–93.

    For an empirical rebuttal to this article, see Bluming, AZ. Breast cancer and hormone-replacement therapy. N Engl J Med 1995 Nov 16;333(20):1357.
21. Sellers TA, Mink PJ, Ceerhan JR, et al. The role of hormone replacement therapy and the risk for breast cancer and total mortality in women with a family history of breast cancer. Ann Intern Med. 1997;127:973–80.

22. Rebbeck TR, Levin AM, Eisen A, et al. Breast cancer risk after bilateral prophylactic oophorectomy in BRCA1 mutation carriers. J Natl Cancer Inst. 1999;91:1475–79.

Rebbeck TR, Friebel T, Wagner T, et al. Effect of short-term hormone replacement therapy on breast cancer risk reduction after bilateral prophylactic oophorectomy in BRCA1 and BRCA2 mutation carriers: The PROSE Study Group. J Clin Oncol. 2005;23:7804–10.

23. Eisen A, Lubinski J, Gronwald J, et al. Hormone therapy and the risk of breast cancer in BRCA1 mutation carriers. J Natl Cancer Inst. 2008;100:1361–67.

24. Kotsopoulos J, Huzarski T, Gronwald J, et al. Hormone replacement therapy after menopause and risk of breast cancer in BRCA1 mutation carriers: A case-control study. Breast Cancer Res Treat. 2016;155:365–73.

25. Consensus Development Conference: Prophylaxis and treatment of osteoporosis. BMJ. 1987;295:914–15.

26. Martin KA, Freeman MW. Postmenopausal hormone replacement therapy. N Engl J Med. 1993;328:1115–17.

27. Bergkvist L, Adami HO, Persson I, et al. The risk of breast cancer after estrogen and estrogen-progestin replacement. N Engl J Med. 1989;321:393–97.

28. Bergkvist L, Adami HO, Persson I, et al. Prognosis after breast cancer diagnosis in women exposed to estrogens and estrogen-progesterone replacement therapy. Am J Epidemiol. 1989;130:221–28.

29. Barrett-Connor E. Postmenopausal estrogen replacement and breast cancer. N Engl J Med. 1989;321:319–20.

30. Estrogen replacement and breast cancer. Harvard Medical School Health Letter. 1989;14(12):1–3.

31. Collaborative Group on Hormonal Factors in Breast Cancer. Breast cancer and hormone replacement therapy: Collaborative reanalysis of data from 51 epidemiological studies of 52,705 women with breast cancer and 108,411 women without breast cancer. Lancet. 1997;350:1047–59.

32. Shapiro S, Farmer RDT, Seaman H, et al. Does hormone replacement therapy cause breast cancer? An application of causal principles to three studies. Part 1. The Collaborative Reanalysis. J Fam Plann Reprod Health Care. 2011;37:103–9.

33. Anderson G. Release of the results of the Estrogen Plus Progestin Trial of the WHI: Data and Safety Monitoring. Press conference remarks. WHI Coordinating Center, July 9, 2002.

    Writing Group for the Women's Health Initiative Investigators. Risk and benefits of estrogen plus progestin in healthy postmenopausal women. Principal results from the Women's Health Initiative randomized controlled trial. JAMA. 2002;288:321–33.

34. Chlebowski RT, Hendrix SL, Langer RD, et al. for the WHI investigators. Influence of estrogen plus progestin on breast cancer and mammography in healthy postmenopausal women: The Women's Health Initiative Randomized Trial. JAMA. 2003;289: 3243–53.

35. Anderson GL, Chlebowski RT, Rossouw JE, et al. Prior hormone therapy and breast cancer risk in the Women's Health Initiative randomized trial of estrogen plus progestin. Maturitas. 2006;55: 103–15.

36. Parker-Pope, Tara, *The Hormone Decision* (Emmaus, PA: Rodale, 2007), 14.

37. Chlebowski RT, Anderson GL, Gass M, et al. Estrogen plus progestin and breast cancer incidence and mortality in postmenopausal women. JAMA. 2010;304:1684–92.

38. Genazzani AR, Gambacciani M. A personal initiative for women's health: To challenge the Women's Health Initiative. Gynecol Endocrinol. 2002;16:255–57.

    Lemay A. The relevance of the Women's Health Initiative results on combined hormone replacement therapy and clinical practice. J Obstet Gynaecol Can. 2002;24:711–15.

    Burger H. Hormone replacement therapy in the post–Women's Health Initiative era. Climacteric. 2003;6:11–36.

39. Shapiro S, de Villers TJ, Pines A, et al. Risks and benefits of hormone therapy: Has medical dogma now been overturned? Climacteric. 2014;17:215–22.

   Shapiro S. Risks of estrogen plus progestin therapy: A sensitivity analysis of the findings in the Women's Health Initiative randomized controlled trial. Climacteric. 2003;6:302–10.

40. Langer RD. The evidence base for HRT: What can we believe? Climacteric. 2017;20:91–96.

41. Parker-Pope, *The Hormone Decision,* 12. The quote is Parker-Pope's report of what Rossouw told her; *high impact* was his term.

42. Rossouw JE. Estrogens for prevention of coronary heart disease: Putting the brakes on the bandwagon. Circulation. 1996;94:2982–85.

43. Chlebowski RT, Aragaki AK. The Women's Health Initiative randomized trials of menopausal hormone therapy and breast cancer: Findings in context. Menopause. 2023;30:454–61.

44. U.S. Cancer Statistics Working Group. U.S. Cancer Statistics Data Visualizations Tool, based on 2022 submission data (1999-2020): U.S. Department of Health and Human Services, Centers for Disease Control and Prevention and National Cancer Institute, November 2023.

45. Antoine C, Ameye L, Paesmans M, et al. Menopausal hormone therapy use in relation to breast cancer incidence in 11 countries. Maturitas. 2016;84:81–88.

46. U.S. Cancer Statistics Working Group, 2023.

47. Doamekpor LA, Head SK, South E, et al. Determinants of hormone replacement therapy knowledge and current hormone replacement therapy use. J Womens Health. 2023;32:283–92.

48. Fournier DV, Weber E, Hoeffken W, et al. Growth rate of 147 mammary carcinomas. Cancer. 1980;45:2198–207.

   Santen RJ, Stuenkel CA, Yue W. Mechanistic effects of estrogens on breast cancer. Cancer J. 2022;28:224–40.

49. Ravdin PM, Cronin KA, Howlander N, Berg CD, Chlebowski RT, et al. The decrease in breast cancer incidence in 2003 in the United States. Reply. N Engl J Med. 2007;356:1670–74.

50. Bluming AZ. A decline in breast-cancer incidence. N Engl J Med. 2007;357:509.

51. Shifren JL, Crandall CJ, Manson JE. Menopausal hormone therapy. JAMA. 2019;321:2458–59.

52. Kuhl H. Is the elevated breast cancer risk observed in the WHI study an artefact? Climacteric. 2004;7:319–22.

    Hodis HN, Sarrel PM. Menopausal hormone therapy and breast cancer: What is the evidence from randomized trials? Climacteric. 2018;21:521–28.

    Bluming AZ, Hodis HN, Langer RD. 'Tis but a scratch: A critical review of the WHI evidence associating menopausal hormone therapy with the risk of breast cancer. Menopause. 2023;30(12): 183–90; https://doi.org/10.1097/GME.0000000000002267.

53. Thomson, Cynthia, and Anderson, Garnet, for the WHI Steering Committee, letter to the editor in response to "Women Have Been Misled About Menopause," *New York Times*, February 26, 2023.

54. Roth JA, Etzioni R, Waters TM, et al. Economic return from the Women's Health Initiative estrogen plus progestin clinical trial. Ann Intern Med. 2014;160:594–602.

55. Sarrel PM, Njike VY, Vinante V, Katz DL. The mortality toll of estrogen avoidance: An analysis of excess deaths among hysterectomized women aged 50 to 59 years. Amer J Pub Health. 2013;103:1583–88.

56. Tang WY, Grothe D, Keshishian A, et al. Pharmacoeconomic and associated cost savings among women who were prescribed systemic conjugated estrogen therapy compared with those without menopausal therapy. Menopause. 2018;25:493–99.

    Sarrel PM. Editorial: Estrogen therapy: economic considerations. Menopause. 2018;25:481–82.

57. Beral V, Million Women Study Collaborators. Breast cancer and hormone-replacement therapy in the Million Women Study. Lancet. 2003;362:419–27.

58. Asilomar Working Group on Recommendations for Reporting of Clinical Trials in the Biomedical Literature. Checklist of information for inclusion in reports of clinical trials. Ann Intern Med. 1996;124:741–43.

    Moher D, Schulz KF, Altman D for the CONSORT Group. The CONSORT statement: Revised recommendations for improving the quality of reports of parallel-group randomized trials. JAMA. 2001;285:1987–91.

    Gigerenzer G, Gaissmaier W, Kurz-Milcke E, et al. Helping doctors and patients make sense of health statistics. Psychol Sci Public Interest. 2008;8:53–96.

59. Individual references for each entry may be found in Bluming AZ, Tavris C. Hormone replacement therapy: Real concerns and false alarms. Cancer J. 2009;15:93–104; and Bluming AZ, Tavris C. What are the real risks for breast cancer? Climacteric. 2012;15: 133–38.

60. Bernstein, Peter L., *Against the Gods: The Remarkable Story of Risk* (New York: John Wiley, 1996), 161.

61. Keating C. The social history of ISIS-2: Triumph and the path not taken. Lancet. 2015;386:e4–e5.

62. ISIS-2 (Second International Study of Infarct Survival) Collaborative Group. Aspirin's effect on myocardial infarct mortality: Randomized trial of intravenous streptokinase, oral aspirin, both or neither among 17,187 cases of suspected acute myocardial infarction. Lancet. 1988;2:349–60.

63. Sleight P. Debate: Subgroup analyses in clinical trials: Fun to look at—but don't believe them! Curr Control Trials Cardiovasc Med. 2000;1:25–27.

64. Colditz et al., The use of estrogens and progestins.

65. Schairer C, Lubin J, Troisi R, et al. Menopausal estrogen and estrogen-progestin replacement therapy and breast cancer risk. JAMA. 2000;283:485–91.

66. Santen RJ, Pinkerton J, McCartney C, et al. Risk of breast cancer with progestins in combination with estrogen as hormone replacement therapy. J Clin Endocrinol Metab. 2001;86:16–23.

67. Henderson BE, Paganini-Hill A, Ross RK. Decreased mortality in users of estrogen replacement therapy. Arch Intern Med. 1991;151:75–78.

    Grodstein F, Stampfer MJ, Colditz GA, et al. Postmenopausal hormone therapy and mortality. N Engl J Med. 1997;336:1769–75.

68. Susser M. What is a cause and how do we know one? A grammar for pragmatic epidemiology. Am J Epidemiol. 1991;133:635–48.

69. Taubes, Gary, "Epidemiology Faces Its Limits", *Science*. 1995;269: 164–69.

70. For one study among very many, see Madsen KM, Hviid A, Vestergaard M, et al. A population-based study of measles, mumps, and rubella vaccination and autism. N Engl J Med. 2002;347: 1477–82. For the larger story of the vaccine hysteria, see Seth Mnookin, *The Panic Virus: A True Story of Medicine, Science, and Fear* (New York: Simon and Schuster, 2011) and Offit, Paul A., *Deadly Choices: How the Anti-Vaccine Movement Threatens Us All* (New York: Basic Books, 2012).

71. Charlton BG. Second thoughts: Attribution of causation in epidemiology: Chain or mosaic? J Clin Epidemiol. 1996;49:105–7.

72. Hill AB. The environment and disease: Association or causation? Proc R Soc Med. 1965;58:295–300.

73. Bush TL, Whiteman M, Flaws JA. Hormone replacement therapy and breast cancer: A qualitative review. Obstet Gynecol. 2001;98:498–508.

74. Henderson IC. Risk factors for breast cancer development. Cancer. 1993;71:2127–40.

Madigan M, Ziegler R, Benichou C, et al. Proportion of breast cancer cases in the United States explained by well-established risk factors. J Natl Cancer Inst. 1995;87:1681–85.

75. Haddow A, Watkinson JM, Paterson E. Influence of synthetic oestrogens upon advanced malignant disease. BMJ. 1944;2:393–98.

76. Massidda B, Mascia V, Broccia G, et al. Estrogen therapy of advanced breast cancer. Minerva Med. 1977;68:2509–16.

77. Mahtani RL, Stein A, Vogel CL. High-dose estrogen as salvage hormonal therapy for highly refractory metastatic breast cancer: A retrospective chart review. Clin Therap. 2009;31:2371–78.

78. Hortobagyi GN, Hug V, Buzdar AU, et al. Sequential cyclic combined hormonal therapy for metastatic breast cancer. Cancer. 1989;64:1002–6.

79. Ingle J, Ahmann D, Green S, et al. Randomized clinical trial of diethylstilbestrol versus tamoxifen in postmenopausal women with advanced breast cancer. N Engl J Med. 1981;304:16–21.

Peethambaram P, Ingle J, Suman V, et al. Randomized clinical trial of diethylstilbestrol versus tamoxifen in postmenopausal women with metastatic breast cancer: An updated analysis. Breast Cancer Res Treat. 1999;54:117–22.

80. Lønning PE, Taylor PD, Anker G, et al. High-dose estrogen treatment in postmenopausal breast cancer patients heavily exposed to endocrine therapy. Breast Cancer Res Treat. 2001;67:111–16.

81. Craig Jordan V, Lewis-Wambi J, Kim H, et al. Exploiting the apoptotic actions of oestrogen to reverse anti-hormonal drug resistance in oestrogen receptor positive breast cancer patients. Breast. 2007;16(Suppl 2):105–13.

Abderrahman B, Craig Jordan V. Estrogen for the treatment and prevention of breast cancer: A tale of 2 Karnovsky lectures. Cancer J. 2022;28:163–68.

82. Mukherjee, Siddhartha, *The Emperor of All Maladies: A Biography of Cancer* (New York: Scribner, 2010), 266.

83. Thun MJ, Hannan LM, Adams-Campbell LL, et al. Lung cancer occurrence in never-smokers: An analysis of 13 cohorts and 22 cancer registry studies. PLoS Med. 2008;5:e185.

84. Centers for Disease Control and Prevention. *U.S. Cancer Statistics Female Breast Cancer Stat Bite.* US Department of Health and Human Services; 2023.

85. Collaborative Group on Hormonal Factors in Breast Cancer. Type and timing of menopausal hormone therapy and breast cancer risk: individual participant meta-analysis of the worldwide epidemiological evidence. Lancet. Aug 29, 2019;394(10204): 1159–68.

86. Powledge, Tabitha M., "Easing Hormone Anxiety," *Scientific American* 297, no. 4 (2007): 32–34.

87. Heiss G, Wallace R, Anderson GL, et al. Health risks and benefits three years after stopping randomized treatment with estrogen and progestin. JAMA. 2008;299:1036–45.

88. Anderson GL, Judd HL, Kauntiz AM, et al. Effects of estrogen plus progestin on gynecologic cancers and associated diagnostic procedures: The Women's Health Initiative randomized trial. JAMA. 2003;290:1739–48.

89. Chlebowski RT, Schwartz AG, Wakelee H, et al. Estrogen plus progestin and lung cancer in postmenopausal women. Lancet. 2009;374:1243–51.

90. Rodriguez C, Feigelson HS, Deka A, et al. Postmenopausal hormone therapy and lung cancer risk in the Cancer Prevention Study II Nutrition Cohort. Cancer Epidemiol Biom Prev. 2008;17:65–60.

    Pesatori AC, Carugno M, Consonni DC, et al. Reproductive and hormonal factors and the risk of lung cancer: The EAGLE study. Int J Cancer. 2013;132:2630–39.

91. Clague J, Reynolds P, Henderson KD, et al. Menopausal hormone therapy and lung cancer–specific mortality following diagnosis: The California Teachers Study. PLoS One. 2014;97: e103735.

Katcoff H, Wenzlaff AS, Schwartz AG. Survival in women with NSCLC: The role of reproductive history and hormone use. J Thorac Oncol. 2014;9:355–61.

92. Hoover R. Hormones in breast cancer: Etiology versus ideology. National Institutes of Health, May 15, 2007; http://videocast.nih .gov/Summary.asp?File=13823.

Chapter 3: Can Breast Cancer Survivors Take Oestrogen?

1. Bluming AZ, Dosik G, Lowitz B, et al. Treatment of primary breast cancer without mastectomy: The Los Angeles community experience and review of the literature. Ann Surg. 1986;204: 136–47.
2. Couzi RJ, Helzsouer KJ, Fetting JH. Prevalence of menopausal symptoms among women with a history of breast cancer and attitudes toward estrogen replacement therapy. J Clin Oncol. 1995;13:2737–44.
3. Hershman DL, Cho C, Crew KD. Management of complications from estrogen deprivation in breast cancer patients. Curr Oncol Rep. 2009;11:29–36.
4. Antoine C, Vandromme J, Fastrez M, et al. A survey among breast cancer survivors: Treatment of the climacteric after breast cancer. Climacteric. 2008;11:322–28.
5. Creasman WT. HRT and women who have had breast or endometrial cancer. J Epidemiol Biostat. 1999;4:217–25.
6. Wile AG, DiSaia PJ. Hormones and breast cancer. Am J Surg. 1989;157:438–42.

DiSaia PJ, Brewster WR, Ziogas A, Anton-Culver H. Breast cancer survival and hormone replacement therapy: A cohort analysis. Am J Clin Oncol. 2000;23:541–45.
7. Huggins C, Moon RC, Morii S. Extinction of experimental mammary cancer. I. Estradiol-17beta and progesterone. PNAS. 1962; 48:379–86.

8. Palshof T, Mouridsen HT, Daehnfeldt JL. Adjuvant endocrine therapy of primary operable breast cancer: Report on the Copenhagen breast cancer trials. Eur J Cancer. 1980;1:183–87.

    Palshof T, Carstensen B, Mouridsen HT, Dombernowsky P. Adjuvant endocrine therapy in pre- and postmenopausal women with operable breast cancer. Rev Endocrine Related Cancer. 1985;17:43–50.

9. Beex L, Pieters PG, Smals A, et al. Tamoxifen versus ethinyl estradiol in the treatment of postmenopausal women with advanced breast cancer. Cancer Treat Rep. 1981;65:179–85.

10. Stoll BA. Effect of Lyndiol, an oral contraceptive, on breast cancer. BMJ. 1967;1:150–53.

11. Baum M. Hormone replacement therapy in breast cancer. Letter to the editor. Lancet. 1994;343:53.

12. Bluming AZ: Hormone replacement therapy: Benefits and risks for the general postmenopausal female population and for women with a history of previously-treated breast cancer. Semin Oncol. 1993;20:662–74.

13. Golden L, Stadel B. Estrogen replacement therapy in breast cancer survivors. Letter to the editor. JAMA. 1995;273:620–21.

14. Bluming AZ. Hormone replacement therapy (HRT) in women with previously treated primary breast cancer: Update XIV. Proc ASCO J Clin Oncol. 2008:15s:20693.

15. Cobleigh MA, Berris RF, Bush T, et al. Estrogen replacement therapy in breast cancer survivors: A time for change. Breast Cancer Committees of the Eastern Cooperative Oncology Group. JAMA. 1994;272:540–45.

16. Verheul HA, Coelingh-Bennick HJ, Kenemans P, et al. Effects of estrogens and hormone replacement therapy on breast cancer risk and on efficacy of breast cancer therapies. Maturitas. 2000;36:1–17.

17. Ylikorkala O, Metsä-Heikkilä M. Hormone replacement therapy in women with a history of breast cancer. Gynecol Endocrinol. 2002;16:469–78.

18. Uršič-Vrščaj M, Bebar S. A case-control study of hormone replacement therapy after primary surgical breast cancer treatment. Eur J Surg Oncol. 1999;25:146–51.

19. Eden JA, Bush T, Nand S, et al. A case-control study of combined continuous estrogen-progestin replacement therapy among women with a personal history of breast cancer. Menopause. 1995;2:67–72.

20. Dew J, Eden J, Beller E, et al. A cohort study of hormone replacement therapy given to women previously treated for breast cancer. Climacteric. 1998;1:137–42.

    Dew JE, Wren BG, Eden JA. Tamoxifen, hormone receptors and hormone replacement therapy in women previously treated for breast cancer: A cohort study. Climacteric. 2002;5:151–55.

21. Durna EM, Wren BG, Heller GZ, et al. Hormone replacement therapy after a diagnosis of breast cancer: Cancer recurrence and mortality. Med J Aust. 2002;177:347–51.

    Durna EM, Heller GZ, Leader LR, et al. Breast cancer in premenopausal women: Recurrence and survival rates and relationship to hormone replacement therapy. Climacteric. 2004;7:284–91.

22. Espie M, Gorins A, Perret F, et al. Hormone replacement therapy (HRT) in patients treated for breast cancer: Analysis of a cohort of 120 patients. Proc ASCO. 1999 (abstract);18:2262.

23. Marttunen MB, Hietanen P, Pyrhonen S, et al. A prospective study on women with a history of breast cancer and with or without estrogen replacement therapy. Maturitas. 2001;39:217–25.

24. Beckmann MW, Jap D, Djahansouzi S, et al. Hormone replacement therapy after treatment of breast cancer: Effects on postmenopausal symptoms, bone mineral density and recurrence rates. Oncol. 2001;60:199–206.

25. Vassilopoulou-Sellin R, Asmar L, Hortobagyi GN, et al. Estrogen replacement therapy after localized breast cancer: Clinical outcome of 319 women followed prospectively. J Clin Oncol. 1999;17:1482–87.

26. Brewster WR, DiSaia PJ, Grosen EA, et al. Experience with estrogen replacement therapy in breast cancer survivors. Int J Fertil Women's Med. 1999;44:186–92.

27. Decker DA, Pettinga JE, Vander Velde N, et al. Estrogen replacement therapy in breast cancer survivors: A matched-controlled series. Menopause. 2003;10:277–85.

28. Peters GN, Fodera T, Sabol J, et al. Estrogen replacement therapy after breast cancer: A 12-year follow-up. Ann Surg Oncol. 2001;8:828–32.

29. O'Meara ES, Rossing MA, Daling JR, et al. Hormone replacement therapy after a diagnosis of breast cancer in relation to recurrence and mortality. J Natl Cancer Inst. 2001;93:754–62.

30. Meurer LN, Lená S. Cancer recurrence and mortality in women using hormone replacement therapy: Meta-analysis. J Fam Pract. 2002;51:1056–62.

31. Ettinger B, Grady D, Tosteson AN, et al. Effect of the Women's Health Initiative on women's decisions to discontinue postmenopausal hormone therapy. Obstet Gynecol. 2003;102:1225–32.

32. Email from Michelle Fujimoto to Avrum Bluming, December 20, 2017. Reprinted with her permission.

33. Letter from Dr. Philip DiSaia to Avrum Bluming, January 3, 2007. Quoted with his permission.

34. Chlebowski RT, Col N. Menopausal hormone therapy after breast cancer. Lancet. 2004;363:410–11.

35. Holmberg L, Anderson H. HABITS (hormonal replacement therapy after breast cancer — is it safe?). A randomized comparison: Trial stopped. Lancet. 2004;363:453–55.

36. Holmberg L, Iversen OE, Rudenstam CM, et al. Increased risk of recurrence after hormone replacement therapy in breast cancer survivors. J Natl Cancer Inst. 2008;100:475–82.

37. Holmberg L, Anderson H. Stopping HABITS. Lancet. 2004;363:1477.

38. Von Schoultz E, Rutqvist LE. Menopausal hormone therapy after breast cancer: The Stockholm randomized trial. J Natl Cancer Inst. 2005;97:533–35.

    For the follow-up, see Fahlén M, Fornander T, Johansson H, et al. Hormone replacement therapy after breast cancer: 10 year follow-up of the Stockholm randomized trial. Eur J Cancer. 2013;49:-52–59.

39. Creasman WT. Hormone replacement therapy after cancers. Curr Opin Oncol. 2005;17:496. Quote is on p. 497.

40. Mueck AO, Rabe T, Kiesel L, Strowitzki T. Hormone replacement therapy after breast cancer. J Reprod Med Endocrinol. 2008;5:83.

41. Society of Obstetricians and Gynecologists of Canada (SOGC). Use of hormonal replacement therapy after treatment of breast cancer. Int J Gynecol Obstet. 2005;88:216–21.

42. Zielinski SL. Hormone replacement therapy for breast cancer survivors: An answered question? J Natl Cancer Inst. 2005;97:955.

43. Garrido-Oyarzún MF, Castelo-Branco C. Use of hormone therapy for menopausal symptoms and quality of life in breast cancer survivors: Safe and ethical? Gynecol Endocrinol. 2017;33:10–15.

44. Bluming AZ. Hormone replacement therapy after breast cancer: It is time. Cancer J. 2022;28:183–90.

45. Col NF, Kim JA, Chlebowski RT. Menopausal hormone therapy after breast cancer: a meta-analysis and critical appraisal of the evidence. Breast Cancer Res. 2005;7:R535–R540.

46. O'Meara et al., Hormone replacement therapy after a diagnosis of breast cancer.

47. Deli T, Orosz M, Jakab A. Hormone replacement therapy in cancer survivors — review of the literature. Pathol Oncol Res. 2020;26:63–78.

48. Poggio F, DelMastro L, Bruzzone M, et al. Safety of systemic hormone replacement therapy in breast cancer survivors: A systematic review and meta-analysis. Breast Cancer Res Treat. 2021;191: 269–75.

49. Batur P, Blixen CE, Moore HCF, et al. Menopausal hormone therapy (HT) in patients with breast cancer. Maturitas. 2006; 53:123–32.

50. Cobleigh MA, Berris RF, Bush T, et al. Estrogen replacement therapy in breast cancer survivors: A time for change. Breast Cancer Committees of the Eastern Cooperative Oncology Group. JAMA. 1994;272:540–45.

51 Winer, Eric, "2023 Presidential Address: Partnering with Patients: The Cornerstone of Clinical Care and Research." *ASCO Connection*, June 6, 2023.

52. Mukherjee, Siddhartha, *The Laws of Medicine: Field Notes from an Uncertain Science* (New York: Simon and Schuster, 2015), 4.

Chapter 4: Matters of the Heart

1. Centers for Disease Control and Prevention. *U.S. Cancer Statistics Female Breast Cancer Stat Bite*. US Department of Health and Human Services; 2023.

2. Assessing the odds. Lancet. 1997;350:1563.

3. Gulati M, Shaw LJ, Merz CNB. Myocardial ischemia in women—lessons from the NHLBI WISE study. Clin Cardiol. 2012;35:141–48.

4. Haukilahti MAE, et al. Sudden cardiac death in women: Causes of death, autopsy findings, and electrocardiographic risk markers. Circ. 2019;139:1012–21.

5. Legato, Marianne J., and Colman, Carol, *The Female Heart: The Truth About Women and Heart Disease* (New York: Perennial Currents, 2000).

    Goldberg, Nieca, *Women Are Not Small Men: Life-Saving Strategies for Preventing and Healing Heart Disease in Women* (New York: Ballantine, 2003).

6. Sinaceur M, Heath C, Cole S. Emotional and deliberative reactions to a public crisis: Mad cow disease in France. Psychol Sci. 2005;16:247–54.

7. Patnaik JL, Byers T, Diguiseppe C, et al. Cardiovascular disease competes with breast cancer as the leading cause of death for older females diagnosed with breast cancer: A retrospective cohort study. Breast Can Res. 2011;13:R64.

8. Quoted in Goodman A, Helwick C. New data on prognostic factors, disease detection, drug toxicities, and treatment adherence presented at SABCS. ASCO Post, February 25, 2017, 18.

9. Mehta LS, Watson KE, Barac C, et al. Cardiovascular disease and breast cancer: Where these entities intersect. A scientific statement from the American Heart Association. Circ. 2018;137:e30–e66.

10. Stampfer MJ, Colditz GA. Estrogen replacement therapy and coronary heart disease: A quantitative assessment of the epidemiologic evidence. Prev Med. 1991;20:47–63.

11. Barrett-Connor E, Bush TL. Estrogen and coronary heart disease in women. JAMA. 1991;265:1861–67. See also Barrett-Connor E, Grady D. Hormone replacement therapy, heart disease, and other considerations. Annu Rev Public Health. 1998;19:55–72.

12. Grodstein F, Manson JE, Colditz GA, et al. A prospective observational study of postmenopausal hormone therapy and primary prevention of cardiovascular disease. Ann Intern Med. 2000;133:933–41.

13. Jacobson BK, Knutson SF, Fraser GE. Age at natural menopause and total mortality and mortality from ischemic heart disease: The Adventist Health Study. J Clin Epidemiol. 1999;52:303–7.

    Rivera CM, Grossardt BR, Rhodes DJ, et al. Increased cardiovascular mortality after early bilateral oophorectomy. Menopause. 2009;16:15–23.

14. Chalmers TC, Celano P, Sacks HS, Smith H Jr. Bias in treatment assignment in controlled clinical trials. N Engl J Med. 1983;309:1358–61.

    Sacks H, Chalmers TC, Smith H Jr. Randomized versus historical controls for clinical trials. Am J Med. 1982;72:233–40.

Colditz GA, Miller JN, Mosteller F. How study design affects outcomes in comparisons of therapy. I. Medical. Stat Med. 1989;8:441–54.

15. Sackett, D. L., et al., *Evidence-Based Medicine: How to Practice and Teach EBM* (New York: Churchill Livingstone, 1997).

16. Concato J, Shah N, Horwitz RI. Randomized, controlled trials, observational studies, and the hierarchy of research designs. N Engl J Med. 2000;342:1887–92.

Steen RG, Dager SR. Evaluating the evidence for evidence-based medicine: Are randomized clinical trials less flawed than other forms of peer-reviewed medical research? FASEB J. 2013;27:3430–36.

Hellman S. Of mice but not men. Problems of the randomized clinical trial. N Engl J Med. 1991;324:1585–89.

17. Benson K, Hartz AJ. A comparison of observational studies and randomized, controlled trials. N Engl J Med. 2000;342:1878–86.

18. Poynard T, Munteanu M, Ratziu V, et al. Truth survival in clinical research: An evidence-based requiem? Ann Intern Med. 2002;136:888–95.

19. Healy, David, *Pharmageddon* (Berkeley: University of California Press, 2012), 95.

20. Rossouw JE, Anderson GL, Prentice RL, et al. Risks and benefits of estrogen plus progestin in healthy postmenopausal women: Principal results from the Women's Health Initiative Randomized Controlled Trial. JAMA. 2002;288:321–33.

21. Speroff L. A clinician's review of the WHI-related literature. Int J Fertil. 2004;49:252–67.

22. Rossouw JE, Prentice RI, Manson JE, et al. Postmenopausal hormone therapy and risk of cardiovascular disease by age and years since menopause. JAMA. 2007;297:1465–77.

23. Grodstein F, Manson JE, Stampfer MJ. Hormone therapy and coronary heart disease: The role of time since menopause and age at hormone initiation. J Women's Health. 2006;15:35–44.

24. Salpeter SR, Walsh JM, Greyber E, et al. Brief report: Coronary heart disease events associated with hormone therapy in younger and older women. A meta-analysis. J Gen Intern Med. 2006;21:363–66.
25. Schierbeck LL, Rejnmark L, Landbo C, et al. Effect of hormone replacement therapy on cardiovascular events and recently post-menopausal women: Randomized trial. BMJ. 2012;345:e6409.
26. Shapiro S. Risks of estrogen plus progestin therapy: A sensitivity analysis of the findings in the Women's Health Initiative randomized controlled trial. Climacteric. 2003;6:302–10.
27. Bhavnani BR, Strickler RC. Menopausal hormone therapy. J Obstet Gynaecol Can. 2005;27:137–62.
28. Hulley S, Grady D, Bush T, et al. Randomized trial of estrogen plus progestin for secondary prevention of coronary heart disease in postmenopausal women. JAMA. 1998;280:605–13.
29. Mikkola TS, Clarkson TB. Estrogen replacement therapy, athero-sclerosis, and vascular function. Cardiovasc Res. 2002;53:605–19.
30. Herrington DM, Reboussin DM, Brosnihan KB, et al. Effects of estrogen replacement on the progression of coronary artery athero-sclerosis. N Engl J Med. 2000;343:522–29.

    Hodis HN, Mack WJ, Lobo RA, et al. Estrogen in the prevention of atherosclerosis. Ann Intern Med. 2001;135:939–53.

    Hodis HN, Collins P, Mack WJ. The timing hypothesis for coronary heart disease prevention with hormone therapy: Past, present and future perspective. Climacteric. 2012;15:217–28.
31. Mikkola TS, Tuomikoski P, Lyytinen H, et al. Increased cardio-vascular mortality risk in women discontinuing postmenopausal hormone therapy. J Clin Endocrinol Metab. 2015;100:4588–94.

    Tuomikoski P, Lyytinen H, Korhonen P, et al. Coronary heart disease mortality and hormone therapy before and after the Women's Health Initiative. Obstet Gynecol. 2014;124:947–53.

32. Hodis HN, Mack WJ, Henderson VW, et al. Vascular effects of early versus late postmenopausal treatment with estradiol. N Engl J Med. 2016;374:1221–31.

33. Parker-Pope, Tara, "How NIH Misread Hormonal Study in 2002," *Wall Street Journal,* July 9, 2007.

34. Kelleher, Susan, and Wilson, Duff, "Suddenly Sick: Change a Number, Create a Patient," special report for the *Seattle Times,* June 26–30, 2005.

35. Olotu BS, Shepherd MD, Novak S, et al. Use of statins and the risk of incident diabetes: A retrospective cohort study. Am J Cardiovasc Drugs. 2016;16:377–90.

    Sattar N, Preiss D, Murray HM, et al. Statins and risk of incident diabetes: A collaborative meta-analysis of randomised statin trials. Lancet. 2010;375:735–42.

36. Roberts, Barbara H., *The Truth about Statins: Risks and Alternatives to Cholesterol-Lowering Drugs* (New York: Pocket Books, 2012). See also Harriet Rosenberg and Danielle Allard, "Evidence for Caution: Women and Statin Use," Women and Health Protection report, 2007, 1-36, available from the Canadian Women's Health Network at https://whp-apsf.ca/pdf/statinsEvidenceCau tion.pdf.

37. Walsh JME, Pignone M. Drug treatment of hyperlipidemia in women. JAMA. 2004;291:2243–52.

38. Petretta M, Costanzo P, Perrone-Filardi P, et al. Impact of gender in primary prevention of coronary heart disease with statin therapy: A meta-analysis. Int J Cardiol. 2010;138:25–31.

    Brugts JJ, Yetgin T, Hoeks SE, et al. The benefits of statins in people without established cardiovascular disease but with cardiovascular risk factors: Meta-analysis of randomized controlled trials. Br Med J. 2009;338:b2376.

39. Redberg RF, Katz MH. Statins for primary prevention: The debate is intense, but the data are weak. JAMA. 2016;316:1979–81.

Yusuf S, Bosch J, Dagenais G, et al. Cholesterol lowering in intermediate-risk persons without cardiovascular disease. New Engl J Med. 2016;374:2021–31.

40. Bonds DE, Lasser N, Qi L, et al. The effect of conjugated equine oestrogen on diabetes incidence: The Women's Health Initiative randomized trial. Diabetologia 2006;49:459–468.

Margolis KL, Bonds DE, Rodabough RJ, et al. Effect of oestrogen plus progestin on the incidence of diabetes in postmeno-pausal women: Results from the Women's Health Initiative hor-mone trial. Diabetologia. 2004;47:1175–87.

Kanaya AM, Herrington D, Vettinghoff E, et al. Glycemic effects of postmenopausal hormone therapy: The Heart and Estrogen/progestin Replacement Study. Ann Intern Med. 2003; 138:1–9.

Slopien R, Wender-Ozegowska E, Rogowicz-Frontczak A, et al. Menopause and diabetes: EMAS clinical guide. Maturitas. 2018;117:6–10.

41. Salpeter SR, Walsh JME, Ormiston TM, et al. Meta-analysis: Effect of hormone replacement therapy on components of the met-abolic syndrome in postmenopausal women. Diabetes Obes Metab. 2006;8:538–64.

42. Kannel WB, Hjortland MC, McNamara PM, et al. Menopause and risk of cardiovascular disease: The Framingham study. Ann Intern Med. 1976;85:447–52.

43. Krumholz HM, Seeman TE, Merrill SS, et al. Lack of association between cholesterol and coronary heart disease mortality and morbidity and all-cause mortality in persons older than 70 years. JAMA. 1994;272:1335–40.

44. For a history of how Ancel Keys promoted cholesterol and a high-fat diet as the major culprits in heart disease and how the Ameri-can Heart Association supported that belief in the virtual absence of evidence, see Gary Taubes, *Good Calories, Bad Calories* (New

York: Random House, 2007), and *The Case for Keto* (New York: Knopf, 2020).

45. Dehghan M, Mente A, Zhang X, et al. Associations of fats and carbohydrate intake with cardiovascular disease and mortality in 18 countries from five continents (PURE): A prospective cohort study. Lancet. 2017;390:P2050–62.

46. Siri-Tarino PW, Sun Q, Hu FB, et al. Meta-analysis of prospective cohort studies evaluating the association of saturated fat with cardiovascular disease. Am J Clin Nutr. 2010;91:535–46.

47. Hodis HN, Mack WJ. Menopausal hormone replacement therapy and reduction of all-cause mortality and cardiovascular disease: It is about time and timing. Cancer J. 2022;28:208–23.

48. Gorsky RD, Koplan JP, Peterson HB, et al. Relative risks and benefits of long-term estrogen replacement therapy: A decision analysis. Obstet Gynecol. 1994;83:161–66.

49. Col NF, Eckman MH, Karas RH, et al. Patient-specific decisions about hormone replacement therapy in postmenopausal women. JAMA. 1997;277:1140–47.

50. Arnson Y, et al. Hormone replacement therapy is associated with less coronary atherosclerosis and lower mortality. J Amer Coll Cardiol. 2017;69:1408.

Chapter 5: Breaking Bad

1. Alswat KA. Gender disparities in osteoporosis. J Clin Med Res. 2017;9:382–87.

2. Sing C-W, Lin T-C, Bartholomew S, et al. Global epidemiology of hip fractures: Secular trends in incidence rate, post-fracture treatment, and all-cause mortality. J Bone Min Res. 2023;38:-1064–75.

3. Cummings SR, Nevitt MC, Browner WS, et al. Risk factors for hip fracture in white women. N Engl J Med. 1995;332:767–74.

4. Brauer CA, Coca-Perraillon M, Cutler DM, et al. Incidence and mortality of hip fractures in the United States. JAMA. 2009;302: 1573–79.

   Goldacre MJ, Roberts SE, Yeates D. Mortality after admission to hospital with fractured neck of femur: Database study. BMJ. 2002;325:868–69.

5. Vestergaard P, Rejnmark L, Mosekilde L. Increased mortality in patients with a hip fracture—effect of pre-morbid conditions in post-fracture complications. Osteoporos Int. 2007;18:1583–93.

   Vestergaard P, Rejnmark L, Mosekilde L. Loss of life years after a hip fracture: Effects of age and sex. Acta Orthopaedica. 2009; 80:525–30.

6. Empana JP, Dargent-Molina P, Béart G, et al. Effect of hip fracture on mortality in elderly women: The EPIDOS prospective study. J Am Geriatr Soc. 2004;52:685–90.

7. Von Friesendorff M, McGuigan FE, Wizert A, et al. Hip fracture, mortality risk, and cause of death over two decades. Osteoporos Int. 2016;27:2945–53.

8. Panula J, Pihlajamäki H, Mattila VM, et al. Mortality and cause of death in hip fracture patients aged 65 or older: A population-based study. BMC Musculoskelet Disord. 2011;12:105; https://bmcmusculoskeletdisord.biomedcentral.com/articles/10.1186/1471-2474-12-105.

9. Seeman E, Delmas PD. Bone quality—the material and structural basis of bone strength and fragility. N Engl J Med. 2006; 354:2250–61.

10. Albright F, Bloomberg E, Smith PH. Post-menopausal osteoporosis. Trans Assoc Am Physicians. 1940;55:298–305.

   Albright F, Burnett CH, et al. Osteomalacia and late rickets: The various etiologies met in the United States with emphasis on that resulting from a specific form of renal acidosis, the therapeutic indications for each etiological sub-group, and the relationship between osteomalacia and Milkman's syndrome. Medicine. 1946;25: 399–479.

Gordan GS. Estrogen and postmenopausal osteoporosis. Ann Intern Med. 1993;118:155.

Henneman PH, Wallach S. A review of the prolonged use of estrogens and androgens in postmenopausal and senile osteoporosis. AMA Arch Intern Med. 1957;100:715–23.

11. Zhao J-G, Zeng X-T, Wang J, et al. Association between calcium or vitamin D supplementation and fracture incidence in community-dwelling older adults: A systematic review and meta-analysis. JAMA. 2017;318:2466–82.

Thomson CA, Aragaki AK, Prentice RL, et al. Long-term effect of randomization to calcium and vitamin D supplementation on health in older women: Postintervention follow-up of a randomized clinical trial. Ann Intern Med 2024;doi:10.7326/M23-2598.

12. Bischoff-Ferrari HA, Dawson-Hughes B, Baron JA, et al. Calcium intake and hip fracture risk in men and women: A meta-analysis of prospective cohort studies and randomized controlled trials. Am J Clin Nutr. 2007;86:1780–90.

13. Jackson RD, LaCroix AZ, Gass M, et al. Calcium plus vitamin D supplementation and the risk of fractures. N Engl J Med. 2006;354:669–83.

14. LeBoff MS, Chou SH, Ratliff KA, et al. Supplemental vitamin D and incident fractures in midline in older adults. N Engl J Med. 2022;387:299–309.

15. Szabo, Liz, "Vitamin D, the Sunshine Supplement, Has Shadowy Money Behind It," *New York Times,* August 18, 2018.

16. Nachtigall LE, Nachtigall RH, Nachtigall RD, et al. Estrogen replacement. I. A 10-year prospective study in the relationship to osteoporosis. Obstet Gynecol. 1979;53:277–81.

Christiansen C, Christiansen MA, Transol I. Bone mass in postmenopausal women after withdrawal of oestrogen/progestogen replacement therapy. Lancet. 1981;1:459–61.

Lobo RA, McCormick W, Singer F, et al. Depomedroxy-progesterone acetate compared with conjugated estrogens for the treatment of postmenopausal women. Obstet Gynecol. 1984; 63:1–5.

17. Peck WA, Barrett-Connor E, Buckwalter JA, et al. Consensus conference: Osteoporosis. JAMA. 1984;252:799–802.

Consensus Development Conference: Prophylaxis and treatment of osteoporosis. BMJ. 1987;295:914–15.

18. Weiss NS, Ure CL, Ballard JH, et al. Decreased risk of fractures of the hip and lower forearm with postmenopausal use of estrogen. N Engl J Med. 1980;303:1195–98.

Kiel DP, Felson DT, Anderson JJ, et al. Hip fracture and the use of estrogens in postmenopausal women: The Framingham study. N Engl J Med. 1987;317:1169–74.

19. Naessén T, Persson I, Adami HO, et al. Hormone replacement therapy and the risk for first hip fracture. A prospective, population-based cohort study. Ann Intern Med. 1990;113:95–103.

Michaëlsson K, Baron JA, Farahmand BY, et al. Hormone replacement therapy and risk of hip fracture: Population-based case-controlled study. BMJ. 1998;316:1858–63.

Von Friesendorff et al. Hip fracture, mortality risk.

20. Rossouw JE, Anderson GL, Prentice RL, et al. Risks and benefits of estrogen plus progestin in healthy postmenopausal women: Principal results from the Women's Health Initiative Randomized Controlled Trial. JAMA. 2002;288:321–33.

Cauley JA, Robbins J, Chen Z, et al. Effects of estrogen plus progestin on risk of fracture and bone mineral density: The Women's Health Initiative Randomized Trial. JAMA. 2003;290:1929–38.

Manson JE, Chlebowski RT, Stefanick ML, et al. The Women's Health Initiative Hormone Therapy Trials: Update and overview of health outcomes during the intervention and post-stopping phases. JAMA. 2013;310:1353–68.

21. Rozenberg S., Vandromme J, Revercez P, et al. Menopause hormone therapy in the management of postmenopausal osteoporosis. Cancer J. 2022;28:204–7.

22. Col, NF, Bowlby LA, McGarry K. The role of menopausal hormone therapy in preventing osteoporotic fractures: A critical review of the clinical evidence. Minerva Med. 2005;96:331–42.

23. Lindsay R, Hart DM, MacLean A, et al. Bone response to termination of oestrogen treatment. Lancet. 1978;1:1325–27.

24. Grady D, Rubin SM, Petitti DB, et al. Hormone therapy to prevent disease and prolong life in postmenopausal women. Ann Intern Med. 1992;117:1016–37.

25. Ettinger B, Grady D. The waning effect of postmenopausal estrogen therapy on osteoporosis. N Engl J Med. 1993;329:1192–93.

26. See mayoclinic.org on osteoporosis: https://www.mayoclinic.org/diseases-conditions/osteoporosis/diagnosis-treatment/drc-20351974.

27. Grob, Gerald N., *Aging Bones: A Short History of Osteoporosis* (Baltimore: Johns Hopkins University Press, 2014), xv.

28. Chestnut CH. Theoretical overview: Bone development, peak bone mass, bone loss, and fracture risk. Am J Med. 1991;91:2S–4S.

    Eisman JA, Sambrook PN, Kelly PJ, et al. Exercise and its interaction with genetic influences in the determination of bone mineral density. Am J Med. 1991;91:5S–9S.

29. Riggs BL, Hodgson SF, O'Fallon WM, et al. Effect of fluoride treatment on the fracture rate in postmenopausal women with osteoporosis. N Engl J Med. 1990;322:802–9.

    Heaney RP. Bone mass, bone fragility, and the decision to treat. JAMA. 1998;280:2119–20.

    Heaney RP, Recker RR. Combination and sequential therapy for osteoporosis. N Engl J Med. 2005;353:624–25.

30. For example, John A. Kanis, a leading British authority, noted that all definitions of osteoporosis based on bone density were arbitrary and that other factors contributed to bone fragility. See Kanis JA. Osteoporosis and osteopenia. J Bone Miner Res. 1990;5:209–10.

31. Grob, *Aging Bones*. See also Grob G., From aging to pathology: The case of osteoporosis. J Hist Med Allied Sci. 2010:1–39.

32. Ettinger B, Miller P, McClung MR. Use of bone densitometry results for decisions about therapy for osteoporosis. Ann Int Med. 1996;125:623.
33. Cheung AM, Detsky AS. Osteoporosis and fractures. Missing the bridge? JAMA. 2008;299:1468–70.
34. Foreman, Judy, "Should Bone Loss Always Be Treated?," *Los Angeles Times,* June 13, 2005.
35. Quoted in Gerald N. Grob and Allan V. Horwitz, *Diagnosis, Therapy, and Evidence: Conundrums in Modern American Medicine* (New Brunswick, NJ: Rutgers University Press, 2010), 195.
36. Tella SH, Gallagher JC. Prevention and treatment of postmenopausal osteoporosis. J Steroid Biochem Mol Biol. 2014;142: 155–70.
37. Wang Z, Ward MM, Chan L, Bhattacharyya T. Adherence to oral bisphosphonates and the risk of subtrochanteric and femoral shaft fractures among female Medicare beneficiaries. Osteoporos Int. 2014;25:2109–16.
38. Odvina C, Zerwekh J, Rao D, et al. Severely suppressed bone turnover: A potential complication of alendronate therapy. J Clin Endocrinol Metab. 2005;90:1294–1301.

Saita Y, Ishijima M, Kaneko K. Atypical femoral fractures and bisphosphonate use: Current evidence and clinical implications. Ther Adv Chron Dis. 2015;6:185–93.

Kharwadkar N, Mayne B, Lawrence JE, et al. Bisphosphonates and atypical subtrochanteric fractures of the femur. Bone Joint Res. 2017;6:144–53.

Schilcher J, Koeppen V, Aspenberg P. Risk of atypical femoral fracture during and after bisphosphonate use. N Engl J Med. 2014;371:974–76.

Shane E, Burr D, Abrahamsen B, et al. Atypical subtrochanteric and diaphyseal femoral fractures: Second report of a task force of the American Society for Bone and Mineral Research. J Bone Miner Res. 2014;29:1–23.

Meier RPH, Perneger TV, Stern R, et al. Increasing occurrence of atypical femoral fractures associated with bisphosphonate use. Arch Intern Med. 2012;172:930–36.

39. Drieling RL, LaCroix AZ, Beresford SAA, et al. Long-term oral bisphosphonate therapy and fractures in older women: The Women's Health Initiative. J Am Geriatr Soc. 2017;65:1924–31.

40. Langer RD, Simon JA, Pines A, et al. Menopausal hormone therapy for primary prevention: Why the USPSTF is wrong. Climacteric. 2017;20:402–13.

41. Ettinger B, Black DM, Mitlak BH, et al. Reduction of vertebral fracture risk in postmenopausal women with osteoporosis treated with raloxifene: Results from a three-year randomized clinical trial. JAMA. 1999;282:637–45; erratum JAMA. 1999;282:2124.

    Grady D, Ettinger B, Moscarelli E, et al. Multiple outcomes of raloxifene evaluation investigators. Safety and adverse effects associated with raloxifene: Multiple outcomes of raloxifene evaluation. Obstet Gynecol. 2004;104:837–44.

    Gambacciani M, Levancini M. Hormone replacement therapy and the prevention of postmenopausal osteoporosis. Prz Menopauzalny. 2014;13:213–20.

42. Silverman SL. Calcitonin. Endocrinol Metab Clin North Amer. 2003;32:273–84.

    Watts NB, Worley K, Solis A, et al. Comparison of risedronate to alendronate and calcitonin for early reduction of nonvertebral fracture risk: Results from a managed care administrative claims database. J Manag Care Pharm. 2004;10:142–51.

    Kung AW, Pasion EG, Sofiyan M, et al. A comparison of teriparatide and calcitonin therapy in postmenopausal Asian women with osteoporosis: A 6-month study. Curr Med Res Opin. 2006;22:929–37.

43. Eriksen DR, Keaveny TM, Gallagher ER, et al. Literature review: The effects of teriparatide therapy at the hip in patients with osteoporosis. Bone. 2014;67:246–56.

44. Brent MB. Abaloparatide: A review of preclinical and clinical studies. Europ J Pharmacology. 2021;909:174409.

Miller PD, Hattersley G, Riis BJ, et al. Effect of abaloparatide vs. placebo on new vertebral fractures in postmenopausal women with osteoporosis: A randomized clinical trial. JAMA. 2016;316:722–33.

45. Qi W-X, Lin F, He A-N. Incidence and risk of denosumab-related hypocalcemia in cancer patients: A systematic review and pooled analysis of randomized controlled studies. Curr Med Res Opin. 2013;29:1067–73.

46. Saag KG, Peterson J, Brandi ML, et al. Romosozumab or alendronate for fracture prevention in women with osteoporosis. N Engl J Med. 2017;377:1417–27.

Rosen CJ. Romosozumab—promising or practice changing? N Engl J Med. 2017;377:1479–80.

47. Taylor, Nick Paul, "Safety Scare Prompts FDA to Reject Amgen's Romosozumab," *Fierce Biotech,* July 17, 2017.

48. Poutoglidou F, Samoladas E, Raikos N, et al. Efficacy and safety of anti-sclerostin antibodies in the treatment of osteoporosis: A meta-analysis and systematic review. J Clinical Densitometry. 2022;25:401–15.

Chapter 6: Losing and Using Our Minds

1. All of the statistics about Alzheimer's are found in Alzheimer's Association, *2023 Alzheimer's Disease Facts and Figures.* Alzheimer's Dement 2023;19(4).

2. Zandi PP, Carlson MC, Plassman BL, et al. Hormone replacement therapy and incidence of Alzheimer disease in older women: The Cache County Study. JAMA. 2002;288:2123–29.

3. Shumaker SA, Legault C, Rapp SR, et al. Estrogen plus progestin and the incidence of dementia and mild cognitive impairment in postmenopausal women: The Women's Health Initiative Memory Study. A randomized controlled trial. JAMA. 2003;289:2651–62.

4. Ibid., 2660.
5. Shumaker SA, Legault C, Kuller L, et al. Conjugated equine estrogens and incidence of probable dementia and mild cognitive impairment in postmenopausal women: Women's Health Initiative Memory Study. JAMA. 2004;291:2947–58.
6. Schneider LS. Estrogen and dementia: Insights from the Women's Health Initiative Memory Study. JAMA. 2004;291:3005–7.
7. Espeland MA, Rapp SR, Shumaker SA, et al. Conjugated equine estrogens and global cognitive function in postmenopausal women: Women's Health Initiative Memory Study. JAMA. 2004;291: 2959–68.
8. Speroff, L. A clinician's review of the WHI-related literature. Int J Fertil. 2004;49:252–67.
9. Simpkins JW, Singh M, for the CARPE group. Consortium for the Assessment of Research on Progestins and Estrogens: Letter to the Editor. J Women's Health. 2004;13:1165–68.

   Wickelgren I. Estrogen research: Brain researchers try to salvage estrogen treatments. Science. 2003;302:1138–39.

   Simpkins JM, Singh M. More than a decade of estrogen neuroprotection. Alzheimer's Dement. 2008;4:S131–36.
10. Shumaker et al., Estrogen plus progestin and the incidence of dementia.
11. Bhavnani BR, Strickler RC. Menopausal hormone therapy. J Obstet Gynaecol Can. 2005;27:137–62.
12. Espeland et al., Conjugated equine estrogens and global cognitive function.
13. Marriott LK, Wenk GL. Neurobiological consequences of long-term estrogen therapy. Curr Dir Psychol Sci. 2004;13:173–76.
14. Arevalo MA, Azcoitia I, Garcia-Segura LM. The neuroprotective actions of oestradiol and oestrogen receptors. Nat Rev Neurosci. 2015;16:17–29.

   Jones KJ. Steroid hormones and neurotrophism: Relationship to nerve injury. Metab Brain Dis. 1988;3:1–16.

Gould E, Woolley CS, Frankfurt M, et al. Gonadal steroids regulate dendritic spine density in hippocampal pyramidal cells in adulthood. J Neurosci. 1990;10:1286–91.

Sherwin BB. Hormones and the brain. J Obstet Gynaecol Can. 2001;23:1102–4.

15. Squire L. Memory in the hippocampus: A synthesis from findings with rats, monkeys, and humans. Psychol Rev. 1992;99: 195–231.

Shughrue PJ, Lane MV, Merchenthaler I. Comparative distribution of estrogen receptor-alpha and -beta mRNA in the rat central nervous system. J Comp Neurol. 1997;388:507–25.

Maki PM, Henderson VW. Hormone therapy, dementia, and cognition: The Women's Health Initiative ten years on. Climacteric. 2012;15:256–62.

16. Opendak M, Briones BA, Gould E. Social behavior, hormones and adult neurogenesis. Front Neuroendocrinol. 2016;41:71–86.

17. Gould et al., Gonadal steroids regulate dendritic spine density.

18. Woolley CS, Wenzel HJ, Schwartzkroin PA. Estradiol increases the frequency of multiple synapse boutons in the hippocampal CA1 region of the adult female rat. J Comp Neurol. 1996;373: 108–17.

Brinton, RD, "Biochemistry of Learning and Memory," in J. L. Martinez and R. B. Kesner, eds., *Learning and Memory: A Biological View* (San Diego: Academic Press, 1991), 199–246.

Singh M, Meyer EM, Millard WJ, et al. Ovarian steroid deprivation results in a reversal learning impairment and compromised cholinergic function in female Sprague Dawley rats. Brain Res. 1994;644:305–12.

Simpkins JW, Green PS, Gridley KE, et al. Role of estrogen replacement therapy and memory enhancement and the prevention of neuronal loss associated with Alzheimer's disease. Am J Med. 1997;103:19S–25S.

Wise P, Smith M, Dubal D, et al. Neuroendocrine influences and repercussions of the menopause. Endocr Rev. 1999;20: 243–48.

Zhao L, Mao Z, Chen S, et al. Early Intervention with an estrogen receptor β-selective phytoestrogenic formulation prolongs survival, improves spatial recognition memory, and slows progression of amyloid pathology in a female mouse model of Alzheimer's disease. J Alzheimer's Dis. 2013;37:403–19.

19. Brinton RD. 17 beta estradiol induction of filopodial growth and cultured hippocampal neurons within minutes of exposure. Mol Cell Neurosci. 1993;4:36–46.

Brinton RD. Estrogen-induced plasticity from cells to circuits: Predictions for cognitive function. Trends Pharmacol. 2009;30: 212–22.

McEwen B, Alves S. Estrogen actions in the central nervous system. Endocr Rev. 1999;20:279–307.

20. Bartus RT, Dean RL, Beer B, et al. The cholinergic hypothesis of memory dysfunction. Science. 1982;217:408–17.

Luine VN. Estradiol increases choline acetyltransferase activity in specific basal forebrain nuclei and projection areas of female rats. Exp Neurol. 1985;89:484–90.

21. Brinton RD, Proffitt P, Tran J, et al. Equilin, a principal component of the estrogen replacement therapy Premarin, increases the growth of cortical neurons via an NMDA receptor-dependent mechanism. Exp Neurol. 1997;147:211–20.

Bhavnani, Strickler, Menopausal hormone therapy. J Obstet Gynaecol Can. 2005;27:137–62.

22. Brinton RD, Chen S, Montoya M, et al. The Women's Health Initiative estrogen replacement therapy is neurotrophic and neuroprotective. Neurobiol of Aging. 2000;21:475–96.

Horsburgh K, Mhairi Macrae I, Carswell H. Estrogen is neuroprotective via an apolipoprotein E–dependent mechanism in a mouse model of global ischemia. J Cereb Blood Flow Metab. 2002;22:1189–95.

Nilsen J, Brinton R. Mechanism of estrogen-mediated neuroprotection: Regulation of mitochondrial calcium and Bcl-2 expression. Proc Natl Acad Sci USA. 2003;100:2842–47.

23. Toran-Allerand CD. The estrogen/neurotrophin connection during neural development: Is co-localization of estrogen receptors with the neurotrophins and their receptors biologically relevant? Dev Neurosci. 1996;18:36–48.

24. Xu H, Gouras GK, Greenfield JP, et al. Estrogen reduces neuronal generation of Alzheimer beta-amyloid peptides. Nat Med. 1998;4:447–51.

McEwen, Alves, Estrogen actions.

Brinton RD. Investigative models for determining hormone therapy–induced outcomes in brain: Evidence in support of a healthy cell bias of estrogen action. Ann NY Acad Sci. 2005;1052:57–74.

25. Alvarez-de-la-Rosa M, Silva I, Nilsen J, et al. Estradiol prevents neural tau hyperphosphorylation characteristic of Alzheimer's disease. Ann NY Acad Sci. 2005;1052:210–24.

26. Dhandapani KM, Brann DW. Estrogen-astrocyte interactions: Implications for neuroprotection. BMC Neurosci. 2002;3:6.

Arevalo et al., The neuroprotective actions.

Norbury R, Cutter WJ, Compton J, et al. The neuroprotective effects of estrogen on the aging brain. Exp Gerontol. 2003;38: 109–17.

27. Sherwin BB. Hormones and the brain. J Obstet Gynaecol Can. 2001;23:1102–4.

Sherwin BB. Estrogen and cognitive functioning in women: Lessons we have learned. Behav Neurosci. 2012;126:123–27.

Shah S, Bell RJ, Davis SR. Homocysteine, estrogen and cognitive decline. Climacteric. 2006;9:77–87.

28. Greene RA. Estrogen and cerebral blood flow: A mechanism to explain the impact of estrogen on the incidence and treatment of Alzheimer's disease. Int J Fertil Women's Med. 2000;45:253–57.

29. Brinton, Estrogen-induced plasticity.

30. Resnick SM, Henderson VW. Hormone therapy and risk of Alzheimer's disease: A critical time. JAMA. 2002;288:2170–72.

   Resnick SM, Maki PM, Rapp SR, et al. Effects of combination estrogen plus progestin hormone treatment on cognition and affect. J Clin Endocrinol Metab. 2006;91:1802–10.

31. Carpenter, Siri, "Does Estrogen Protect Memory?," *American Psychological Association Monitor* (January 2001): 52.

32. Caldwell BM, Watson RI. An evaluation of psychological effects of sex hormone administration in aged women: Results of therapy after six months. J Gerontol. 1952;7:228–44.

33. Kantor HI, Michael CM, Shore H. Estrogen for older women. Am J Obstet Gynecol. 1973;116:115–18.

34. Sherwin BB. Estrogen and/or androgen replacement therapy and cognitive functioning in surgically menopausal women. Psychoneuroendocrinol. 1988;13:345–57.

35. Chester, B., "Restoring Remembering: Hormones and Memory," *McGill Reporter,* February 8, 2001.

36. Phillips SM, Sherwin BB. Effects of estrogen on memory function in surgically menopausal women. Psychoneuroendocrinol. 1992; 17:485–95.

37. Sherwin BB, Tulandi T. "Add-back" estrogen reverses cognitive deficits induced by a gonadotropin-releasing hormone agonist in women with leiomyomata uteri. J Clin Endocrinol Metab. 1996;81:2545–49.

   Kampen DL, Sherwin BB. Estrogen use and verbal memory in healthy postmenopausal women. Obstet Gynecol. 1994;83:979–83.

   Kimura D. Estrogen replacement therapy may protect against intellectual decline in postmenopausal women. Horm Behav. 1995;29:312–21.

38. Matyi JM, Rattinger GB, Schwartz S, et al. Lifetime estrogen exposure and cognition in late life: The Cache County Study. Menopause. 2019;26:1366–74.
39. Paganini-Hill A, Henderson VW. Estrogen replacement therapy and risk of Alzheimer disease. Arch Intern Med. 1996;156:2213–17.
40. Tang MX, Jacobs D, Stern Y, et al. Effect of oestrogen during menopause on risk and age at onset of Alzheimer's disease. Lancet. 1996;348:429–32.
41. Baldereschi M, DiCarlo A, Lepore V, et al. Estrogen replacement therapy and Alzheimer's disease in the Italian Longitudinal Study on Aging. Neurol. 1998;50:996–1002.
42. Bagger YZ, Tanko LB, Alexandersen P, et al. for the PERF Study Group. Early postmenopausal hormone therapy may prevent cognitive impairment later in life. Menopause. 2005;12:12–17.
43. Hogervorst E, Williams J, Budge M, et al. The nature of the effect of female gonadal hormone replacement therapy on cognitive function in post-menopausal women: A meta-analysis. Neurosci. 2000;101:485–512.

    LeBlanc ES, Janowsky J, Chan BKS, et al. Hormone replacement therapy and cognition: Systemic review and meta-analysis. JAMA. 2001;285:1489–99.

    Maki PM, Dennerstein L, Clark M, et al. Perimenopausal use of hormone therapy is associated with enhanced memory and hippocampal function later in life. Brain Res. 2011;1379:232–43.
44. Paganini-Hill A, Ross RK, Henderson BE. Postmenopausal oestrogen treatment and stroke: A prospective study. BMJ. 1988;297:519–22.

    Hunt K, Vessey M, McPherson K. Mortality in a cohort of long-term users of hormone replacement therapy: An updated analysis. Br J Obstet Gynaecol. 1990;97:1080–86.

    Finucane FF, Madans JH, Bush TL, et al. Decreased risk of stroke among postmenopausal hormone users: Results from a national cohort. Arch Intern Med. 1993;153:73–79.

Falkeborn M, Persson I, Terent A, et al. Hormone replacement therapy and the risk of stroke: Follow-up of a population-based cohort in Sweden. Arch Intern Med. 1993;153:1201–9.

45. Boysen G, Nyboe J, Appleyard M, et al. Stroke incidence and risk factors for stroke in Copenhagen, Denmark. Stroke. 1988;19: 1345–53.

Pedersen AT, Lidegaard O, Kreiner S, et al. Hormone replacement therapy and risk of non-fatal stroke. Lancet. 1997;350: 1277–83.

Petitti DB, Sidney S, Quesenberry CP Jr., et al. Ischemic stroke and use of estrogen and estrogen/progestogen as hormone replacement therapy. Stroke. 1998;29:23–28.

46. Wilson PW, Garrison RJ, Castelli WP. Postmenopausal estrogen use, cigarette smoking, and cardiovascular morbidity in women over 50: The Framingham study. N Engl J Med. 1985;313:1038–43.

Lemaitre RN, Heckbert SR, Psaty BM, et al. Hormone replacement therapy and associated risk of stroke in postmenopausal women. Arch Intern Med. 2002;162:1954–60.

47. Simon JA, Hsia J, Cauley JA, et al. Postmenopausal hormone therapy and risk of stroke: The Heart and Estrogen/Progestin Replacement Study (HERS). Circulation. 2001;103:638–42.

48. Viscoli CM, Brass LM, Kernan WN, et al. A clinical trial of estrogen replacement therapy after ischemic stroke. N Engl J Med. 2001;345:1243–49.

49. Anderson GL, Limacher M, Assaf AR, et al. Effects of conjugated equine estrogen in postmenopausal women with hysterectomy: The Women's Health Initiative Randomized Controlled Trial. JAMA. 2004;291:1701–12.

50. Maclaren K, Stevenson JC. Primary prevention of cardiovascular disease with HRT. Women's Health. 2012:8:63–74.

Stevenson JC, Hodis HN, Pickar JH, et al. Coronary heart disease and menopause management: The swinging pendulum of HRT. Atherosclerosis. 2009;207:336–40.

51. Mastorakos G, Sakkas EG, Xydakis AM, et al. Pitfalls of the WHI's Women's Health Initiative. Ann NY Acad Sci. 2006;1092: 331–40.

52. Birge SJ. Hormone therapy and stroke. Clin Obstet Gynecol. 2008;51:581–91.

53. Boardman HMP, Hartley L, Eisinga A, et al. Hormone therapy for preventing cardiovascular disease in post-menopausal women. Cochrane Database of Systematic Reviews. 2015;3:CD002229.

54. Shao H, Breitner JC, Whitmer RA, et al. Hormone therapy and Alzheimer disease dementia: New findings from the Cache County Study. Neurol. 2012;79:1846–52.

    Whitmer RA, Quesenberry CP Jr., Zhou J, et al. Timing of hormone therapy and dementia: The critical window theory revisited. Ann Neurol. 2011;69:163–69.

55. Brinton, Investigative models for determining hormone therapy–induced outcomes.

56. Sherwin, Hormones and the brain.

57. Sherwin, Estrogen and cognitive functioning.

58. Maki et al., Perimenopausal use of hormone therapy.

    Maki, Henderson. Hormone therapy, dementia, and cognition.

    Henderson VW, Benke KS, Green RC, et al. Postmenopausal hormone therapy and Alzheimer's disease risk: Interaction with age. J Neurol Neurosurg Psychiatry. 2005;76:103–5.

    Henderson VW. Alzheimer's disease: Review of hormone therapy trials and implications for treatment and prevention after menopause. J Steroid Biochem Mol Biol. 2014;142:99–106.

    MacLennan AH, Henderson VW, Paine BJ, et al. Hormone therapy, timing of initiation and cognition in women aged older than 60 years: The REMEMBER pilot study. Menopause. 2006;13:28–36.

59. M. Fox, "Jellyfish Memory Supplement Prevagen Is a Hoax, FTC Says," NBC News, February 7, 2017.

60. Degnan, William J., Barraza, Leila, Farland, Leslie V., et al., "Strengthening the Regulation of Dietary Supplements — Lessons

from Prevagen." Food and Drug Law Institute, Winter 2021. Available at FDLI.org.

61. Ari A, Frölich L, Ballard C, et al. Effect of idalopirdine as adjunct to cholinesterase inhibitor on change in cognition in patients with Alzheimer disease: Three randomized clinical trials. JAMA. 2018;19:13–42.

   Bennett DA. Lack of benefit with idalopirdine for Alzheimer disease: Another therapeutic failure in a complex disease process. JAMA. 2018;19:123–25.

62. Garber, Judith, "A Tale of Two Drugs: Accountability and Evidence in Alzheimer's Treatments." The Lown Institute (lowninstitute.org.), January 20, 2023.

63. Bateman RJ, et al. Two phase 3 trials of gantenerumab in early Alzheimer's disease. N Engl J Med. 2023; https://doi.org/10.1056/NEJMoa2304430.

   Quoted in Putka, Sophie, "Gantenerumab Failed to Slow Cognitive Decline in Early Alzheimer's," MedPage Today, November 15, 2023.

64. Buckley RF, Gong J, Woodward M. A call to action to address sex differences in Alzheimer disease clinical trials. JAMA Neurology. 2023;80:769–70.

65. Answer by Jonathan Graff-Radford at https://www.mayoclinic.org/diseases-conditions/alzheimers-disease/expert-answers/alzheimers-prevention/faq-20058140.

66. Melby-Lervåg M, Redick TS, Hulme C. Working memory training does not improve performance on measures of intelligence or other measures of 'far transfer': Evidence from a meta-analytic review. Perspec Psychol Sci. 2016;11:512–34.

67. Shipstead Z, Hicks KL, Engle RW. Cogmed working memory training: Does the evidence support the claims? J Appl Res Mem Cog. 2012;1:185–93.

68. Redick TS. Working memory training and interpreting interactions in intelligence interventions. Intelligence. 2015;50:14–20.

69. Simons DJ, Boot WR, Charness N, et al. Do "brain-training" programs work? Psychol Sci Public Interest. 2016;17:103–86.

70. Nilsson J, Lebedev AV, Rydström A, et al. Direct-current stimulation does little to improve the outcome of working memory training in older adults. Psychol Sci. 2017;28:907–20.

71. Blondell SJ, Hammersley-Mather R, Veerman JL. Does physical activity prevent cognitive decline and dementia? A systematic review and meta-analysis of longitudinal studies. BMC Public Health. 2014;14:510.

72. Brasure M, Desai P, Davila H, et al. Physical activity interventions in preventing cognitive decline and Alzheimer-type dementia: A systematic review. Ann Intern Med. 2018;168:30–38.

73. Carpenter, "Does Estrogen Protect Memory?"

74. Henderson et al., Prior use of hormone therapy.

75 Nerattini M, Jett S, Andy C, et al. Systematic review and meta-analysis of the effects of menopause hormone therapy on risk of Alzheimer's disease and dementia. Front. Aging Neurosci. 2023:15. 2023. doi.org/10.3389/fnagi.2023.1260427.

76. Pourhadi N, Mørch LS, Holm EA, et al. Menopausal hormone therapy and dementia: Nationwide, nested, case-control study. BMJ. 2023;381:e072770.

77. Kentarci K, Manson JE. Menopausal hormone therapy and dementia. BMJ. 2023;381:1404.

78. Bagger et al., Early postmenopausal hormone therapy.

Chapter 7: Progesterone and the Pill

1. Stefanick ML, Anderson GL, Margolis KL, et al. for the WHI Investigators. Effects of conjugated equine estrogens on breast cancer and mammography screening in postmenopausal women with hysterectomy. JAMA. 2006;295:1647–57.

For the WHI follow-up: Manson JE, Chlebowski RT, Stefanick ML, et al. Menopausal hormone therapy and health outcomes during the intervention and extended poststopping phases of the Women's Health Initiative Randomized Trials. JAMA. 2013;310:1352–68.

2. Roehm E. A reappraisal of Women's Health Initiative estrogen-alone trial: Long-term outcomes in women 50–59 years of age. Obstet Gynecol Int. 2015; article ID 713295.

3. Anderson GL, Limacher M, Assaf AR, et al. Effects of conjugated equine estrogen in postmenopausal women with hysterectomy: The Women's Health Initiative Randomized Controlled Trial. JAMA. 2004;291:1701–12.

   Viscoli CM, Brass LM, Kernan WN, et al. A clinical trial of estrogen replacement therapy after ischemic stroke. N Engl J Med. 2001;345:1243–49.

   Ross RK, Paganini-Hill A, Wan PC, et al. Effect of hormone replacement therapy on breast cancer risk: Estrogen versus estrogen plus progestin. J Natl Cancer Inst. 2000;92:328–32.

   Chen CL, Weiss NS, Newcomb P, et al. Hormone replacement therapy in relation to breast cancer. JAMA. 2002;287:734–41.

   Porch JV, Lee IM, Cook NR, et al. Estrogen-progestin replacement therapy and breast cancer risk: The Women's Health Study. Cancer Causes Control. 2002;13:847–54.

   Weiss LK, Burkman RT, Cushing-Haugen KL, et al. Hormone replacement therapy regimens and breast cancer risk. Obstet Gynecol. 2002;100:1148–58.

   Li CI, Malone KE, Porter PL, et al. Relationship between long durations and different regimens of hormone therapy and risk of breast cancer. JAMA. 2003;289:3254–63.

   Olsson HL, Ingvar C, Bladstrom A. Hormone replacement therapy containing progestogens and given continuously increases breast carcinoma risk in Sweden. Cancer. 2003;97:1387–92.

4. Cowan LD, Gordis L, Tonascia JA, et al. Breast cancer incidence in women with a history of progesterone deficiency. Am J Epidemiol. 1981;114:209–17.

5. Van Veelen H, Willemse PHB, Tjabbes T, et al. Oral high-dose medroxyprogesterone acetate versus tamoxifen: A randomized crossover trial in postmenopausal patients with advanced breast cancer. Cancer. 1986;58:7–13.

   Parazzini F, Colli E, Scatigna M, et al. Treatment with tamoxifen and progestins for metastatic breast cancer in postmenopausal women: A quantitative review of published randomized clinical trials. Oncol. 1993;50:483–89.

6. Badwe R, Hawlader R, Parmar V, et al. Single-injection depot progesterone before surgery and survival in women with operable breast cancer: A randomized controlled trial. J Clin Oncol. 2011;29:2845–51.

   See also Badwe RA, Wang DY, Gregory WM, et al. Serum progesterone at the time of surgery and survival in women and premenopausal operable breast cancer. Eur J Cancer. 1994;30A: 445–48.

7. Strom BL, Berlin JA, Weber AL, et al. Absence of an effect of injectable and implantable progestin-only contraceptives on subsequent risk of breast cancer. Contraception. 2004;69:353–60.

8. Mohammed H, Russell A, Stark R, et al. Progesterone receptor modulates estrogen receptor-α action in breast cancer. *Nature*. 2015;523:313–17.

   Carroll JS, Hickey TE, Tarulli GA, et al. Deciphering the divergent roles of progestogen in breast cancer. Nat Rev Cancer. 2017;17:54–64.

9. Kuhl H, Stevenson J. The effect of medroxyprogesterone acetate on estrogen-dependent risks and benefits—an attempt to interpret the Women's Health Initiative results. Gynecol Endocrinol. 2006;22:303–17.

10. Santen RJ, Pinkerton J, McCartney C, et al. Risk of breast cancer with progestins in combination with estrogen as hormone replacement therapy. J Clin Endocrinol Metab. 2001;86:21.

11. Micheli A, Muti P, Secreto G, et al. Endogenous sex hormones and subsequent breast cancer in pre-menopausal women. Int J Cancer. 2004;112:312–18.

   Berrino F, Muti P, Micheli A, et al. Serum sex hormone levels after menopause and subsequent breast cancer. J Natl Cancer Inst. 1996;88:291–96.

12. Gadducci A, Biglia N, Cosio S, et al. Progestagen component and combined hormone replacement therapy in postmenopausal women and breast cancer risk: A debated clinical issue. Gynecol Endocrinol. 2009;25:807–15.

13. Campagnoli C, Abba C, Ambrogio S, et al. Pregnancy, progesterone and progestins in relation to breast cancer risk. J Steroid Biochem Mol Biol. 2005;97:441–50.

   Campagnoli C, Clavel-Chapelon F, Kaaks R, et al. Progestins and progesterone and hormone replacement therapy and the risk of breast cancer. J Steroid Biochem Mol Biol. 2005;96:95–108.

   Sitruk-Ware R. Progestogens in a hormonal replacement therapy: New molecules, risks, and benefits. Menopause. 2002;9:6–15.

   De Lignières B, de Vathaire F, Fournier S, et al. Combined hormone replacement therapy and risk of breast cancer in a French cohort study of 3175 women. Climacteric. 2002;5:332–40.

   Fournier A, Berrino F, Riboli E, et al. Breast cancer risk in relation to different types of hormone replacement therapy in the E3N-EPIC cohort. Int J Cancer. 2005;114:448–54.

   Fournier A, Berrino F, Clavel-Chapelon F. Unequal risk for breast cancer associated with different hormone replacement therapies: Results from E3N cohort study. Breast Cancer Res Treat. 2008;107:103–11.

   Murkes D, Conner P, Leifland K, et al. Effects of percutaneous estradiol-oral progesterone versus oral conjugated equine estrogens-medroxyprogesterone acetate on breast cell proliferation and Bcl-2 protein in healthy women. Fertil Steril. 2011;95:1188–91.

14. Siegel RL, Wagle NS, Cercek A, et al. Colorectal cancer statistics, 2023. CA Cancer J Clin. 2023 May–Jun;73(3):233–54.

15. Barzi A, Lenz AM, Labonte MJ, et al. Molecular pathways: Estrogen pathway in colorectal cancer. Clin Cancer Res. 2013;19: 5842–48.

16. Hendifar A, Yang D, Lenz F, et al. Gender disparities in metastatic colorectal cancer survival. Clin Cancer Res. 2009;15:6391–97.

    Fernandez E, Bosetti C, La Vecchia C, et al. Sex differences in colorectal cancer mortality in Europe, 1955–1996. Eur J Cancer Prev. 2000;9:99–104.

    Hildebrand JS, Jacobs EJ, Campbell PT, et al. Colorectal cancer incidence and postmenopausal hormone use by type, recency, and duration in cancer prevention study II. Cancer Epidemiol Biomarkers Prev. 2009;18:2835–41.

    Tannen RL, Weiner MG, Die D, et al. A simulation using data from a primary care practice database closely replicated the Women's Health Initiative trial. J Clin Epidemiol. 2007;60:686–95.

    Rennert G, Rennert HS, Pinchev M, et al. Use of hormone replacement therapy and the risk of colorectal cancer. J Clin Oncol. 2009;27:4542–47.

    Green J, Czanner G, Reeves G, et al. Menopausal hormone therapy and risk of gastrointestinal cancer: Nested case-control study within a prospective cohort, and meta-analysis. Int J Cancer. 2012;130:2387–96.

    Calle EE, Miracle-McMahill HL, Thun MJ, et al. Estrogen replacement therapy and risk of fatal colon cancer in a prospective cohort of postmenopausal women. J Natl Cancer Inst. 1995;87:517–23.

    Slattery ML, Anderson K, Samovitz W, et al. Hormone replacement therapy and improved survival among postmenopausal women diagnosed with colon cancer (USA). Cancer Causes Control. 1999;10:467–73.

Mandelson MT, Miglioretti D, Newcomb PA, et al. Hormone replacement therapy in relation to survival in women diagnosed with colon cancer. Cancer Causes Control. 2003;14:979–84.

Chan JA, Meyerhardt JA, Chan AT, et al. Hormone replacement therapy and survival after colorectal cancer diagnosis. J Clin Oncol. 2006;24:5680–86.

17. Tsilidis KK, Allen NE, Key TJ, et al. Menopausal hormone therapy and risk of colorectal cancer in the European Prospective Investigation into Cancer and Nutrition. Int J Cancer. 2011;128:1881–89.

Newcomb PA, Chia VM, Hampton JM, et al. Hormone therapy in relation to survival from large bowel cancer. Cancer Causes Control. 2009;20:409–16.

18. Hartz A, He T, Ross JJ. Risk factors for colon cancer in 150,912 postmenopausal women. Cancer Causes Control. 2012;23:1599–605.

Hoffmeister M, Raum E, Krtschil A, et al. No evidence for variation in colorectal cancer risk associated with different types of postmenopausal hormone therapy. Clin Pharmacol Ther. 2009;86: 416–24.

19. Vessey MP, Doll R. Investigation of relation between use of oral contraceptives and thromboembolic disease. BMJ. 1968;2: 199–205.

20. Kiley J, Hammond C. Combined oral contraceptives: A comprehensive review. Clin Obstet Gynecol. 2007;50:868–77.

21. Kaunitz AM. Clinical practice: Hormonal contraception in women of older reproductive age. N Engl J Med. 2008;358:1262.

Ratner S, Ofri D. Menopause and hormone-replacement therapy. Part 2. Hormone-replacement therapy regimens. West J Med. 2001; 175(1):32–34.

22. Centers for Disease Control, Cancer and Steroid Hormone Study. Long-term oral contraceptive use and the risk of breast cancer. JAMA. 1983;249:1591–95.

Centers for Disease Control. Oral contraceptive (OC) use and the risk of breast cancer in young women. MMWR. 1984;33:353–54.

Cancer and Steroid Hormone (CASH) Study of the Centers for Disease Control and the National Institute of Child Health and Human Development. Oral-contraceptive use and the risk of breast cancer. N Engl J Med. 1986;315:405–11.

Murray P, Stadel BV, Schlesselman JJ. Oral contraceptive use in women with a family history of breast cancer. Obstet Gynecol. 1989;73:977–83.

23. Marchbanks PA, McDonald JA, Wilson HG, et al. Oral contraceptives and the risk of breast cancer. N Engl J Med. 2002;346: 2025–32.

24. Hannaford PC, Selvaraj S, Elliott AM, et al. Cancer risk among users of oral contraceptives: Cohort data from the Royal College of General Practitioners Oral Contraception Study. BMJ. 2007; 335:651–58.

25. Figueiredo JC, Bernstein L, Capanu M, et al. for the WECARE Study Group. Oral contraceptives, postmenopausal hormones, and risk of asynchronous bilateral breast cancer: The WECARE Study Group. J Clin Oncol. 2008;26:1411–18.

Figueiredo JC, Haile RW, Bernstein L, et al. Oral contraceptives and postmenopausal hormones and risk of contralateral breast cancer among BRCA1 and BRCA2 mutation carriers and non-carriers: The WECARE Study. Breast Cancer Res Treat. 2010;120:175–83.

26. Hunter DJ, Colditz GA, Hankinson SE, et al. Oral contraceptive use and breast cancer: A prospective study of young women. Cancer Epidemiol Biomarkers Prev. 2010;19:2496–502.

27. Moorman PG, Havrilesky LJ, Gierisch JM, et al. Oral contraceptives and risk of ovarian cancer and breast cancer among high-risk women: A systematic review and meta-analysis. J Clin Oncol. 2013;31:4188–98.

28. Vessey MP, Doll R, Jones K, et al. An epidemiological study of oral contraceptives and breast cancer. BMJ. 1979;175:1757–60.

Spencer JD, Millis RR, Hayward JL. Contraceptive steroids and breast cancer. BMJ. 1978;1:1024–26.

Matthews PN, Millis RR, Hayward JL. Breast cancer in women who have taken contraceptive steroids. BMJ. 1981;282: 772–76.

29. American Cancer Society. Key Statistics for Ovarian Cancer, 2024 estimates. Available at cancer.org.

30. Kiley J, Hammond C. Combined oral contraceptives: A comprehensive review. Clin Obstet Gynecol. 2007;50:868–77.

31. Vessey MP, Painter R. Endometrial and ovarian cancer and oral contraceptives—findings in a large cohort study. Br J Cancer. 1995;71:1340–42.

Vessey M, Yeates D, Flynn S. Factors affecting mortality in a large cohort study with special reference to oral contraceptive use. Contraception. 2010;82:221–29.

Bast RC, Brewer M, Zou C, et al. Prevention and early detection of ovarian cancer: Mission impossible? Recent Results Cancer Res. 2007;174:91–100.

Walker GR, Schlesselman JJ, Ness RB. Family history of cancer, oral contraceptive use, and ovarian cancer risk. Obstet Gynecol. 2002;186:8–14.

32. Collaborative Group on Hormonal Factors in Breast Cancer. Breast cancer and hormonal contraceptives: Collaborative reanalysis of individual data on 53,297 women with breast cancer and 100,239 women without breast cancer from 54 epidemiological studies. Lancet. 1996;347:1713–27.

33. ESHRE Capri Workshop Group. Hormones and breast cancer. Hum Reprod Update. 2004;10:281–93.

34. Rabin, Roni Caryn, "Birth Control Pills Still Linked to Breast Cancer, Study Finds," *New York Times,* December 6, 2017.

35. Mørch LS, Skovlund CW, Hannaford PC, et al. Contemporary hormonal contraception and the risk of breast cancer. N Engl J Med. 2017;377:2228–39.

36. Hunter DJ. Oral contraceptives and the small increased risk of breast cancer. N Engl J Med. 2017;377:2276–77.

37. Michels KA, Pfeiffer RM, Brinton LA, et al. Modification of the associations between duration of oral contraceptive use and ovarian, endometrial, breast, and colorectal cancers. JAMA Oncol. 2018;4:516–21.

38. Fitzpatrick D, Pine D, Reeves G, et al. Combined and progestogen-only hormonal contraceptives and breast cancer risk: A UK nested case-control study and meta-analysis. PLoS Medicine. 2023;20: e1004188.

39. Mørch et al., Contemporary hormonal contraception and the risk of breast cancer.

40. Stuenkel C. More evidence why the product labeling for low-dose vaginal estrogen should be changed? Menopause. 2018;25:4–6.

41. Crandall CJ, Hovey KM, Andrews CA, et al. Breast cancer, endometrial cancer, and cardiovascular events in participants who used vaginal estrogen in the Women's Health Initiative Observational Study. Menopause. 2018;25:11–20.

42. McVicker L, Labeit AM, Coupland CAC, et al. Vaginal estrogen therapy use and survival in females with breast cancer. Ann Intern Med. 2024;10:103–8.

Chapter 8: Debates and Final Lessons in the Case for HRT

1. Love, Susan. *Dr. Susan Love's Menopause and Hormone Book* (New York: Random House, 2003), 23.

2. Ravdin's argument may be found here: Ravdin PM, Cronin KA, Howlader N, et al. The decrease in breast cancer incidence in 2003 in the United States. N Engl J Med. 2007;356:1670–74.

3. Ravdin PM, Cronin KA, Chlebowski RT. A decline in breast cancer incidence. N Engl J Med. 2007;357:513. Comment was in response to Bluming AZ. Correspondence: A decline in breast-cancer incidence. Letter to the editor. N Engl J Med. 2007;357:509–13.

4. Anderson GL, Chlebowski RT, Aragaki AK, et al. Conjugated equine oestrogen and breast cancer incidence and mortality in postmenopausal women with hysterectomy: Extended follow-up of the Women's Health Initiative randomised placebo-controlled trial. Lancet Oncol. 2012;13:476–86.

5. Ostrom, Carol M., "Estrogen-Only Pills Cut Breast-Cancer Risk for Some," *Seattle Times,* March 6, 2012.

6. Smyth, Chris, "Women Told Hormone Replacement Therapy Does Not Lead to Early Death," *Times* (UK), September 13, 2017.

7. Manson JE, Aragaki AK, Rossouw JE, et al. Menopausal hormone therapy and long-term all-cause and cause-specific mortality: The Women's Health Initiative Randomized Trials. JAMA. 2017;318:927–38.

8. Sloman, Steven, and Fernbach, Philip, *The Knowledge Illusion: Why We Never Think Alone* (New York: Riverhead Books, 2017), 160.

9. Kahneman, Daniel, *Thinking, Fast and Slow* (New York: Farrar, Straus and Giroux, 2011), 276.

10. Tavris, Carol, and Aronson, Elliot, *Mistakes Were Made (but Not by Me),* Third Ed. (Boston: Mariner, 2020).

11. Tatsioni A, Siontis GCM, Ioannidis JPA. Partisan perspectives in the medical literature: A study of high frequency editorialists favoring hormone replacement therapy. J Gen Intern Med. 2010;25:914–19.

12. Vera-Badillo FE, Shapiro R, Ocana A, et al. Bias in reporting of end points of efficacy and toxicity in randomized, clinical trials for women with breast cancer. Ann Oncol. 2013;24:1238–44.

13. Visvanathan K, Levit LA, Raghavan D, et al. Untapped potential of observational research to inform clinical decision making:

American Society of Clinical Oncology research statement. J Clin Oncol. 2017;35:1845–54.

14. Frieden TR. Evidence for health decision making — beyond randomized, controlled trials. N Engl J Med. 2017;377:465–75.
15. Lobo RA. Hormone replacement therapy: Current thinking. Nat Rev Endocrinol. 2017;13:220–31.
16. U.S. Preventive Services Task Force Recommendation Statement. Hormone therapy for the primary prevention of chronic conditions in postmenopausal women. JAMA. 2017;318:2224–33.
17. The 2017 Hormone Therapy Position Statement of the North American Menopause Society. Menopause. 2017;24:728–53.
18. Santen RJ, Allred DC, Ardoin SP, et al. Postmenopausal hormone therapy: An Endocrine Society scientific statement. J Clin Endocrinol Metab. 2010;95:S1–S6.
19. Erdem U, Ozdegirmenci O, Sobaci E, et al. Dry eye in postmenopausal women using hormone replacement therapy. Maturitas. 2007;56:257–62.

    Schaumberg DA, Buring JE, Sullivan DA, et al. Hormone replacement therapy and dry eye syndrome. JAMA. 2001;286: 2114–19.
20. Edelson RN. Menstrual migraine and other hormonal aspects of migraine. Headache. 1985;25:376–79.
21. Lobo, Hormone replacement therapy.
22. Mehta J, Kling JM, Manson JE. Risks, benefits, and treatment modalities of menopausal hormone therapy: Current concepts. Front Endocrinol. 2021;12;564781.
23. Panay N, Hamoda H, Arya R, et al. The 2013 British Menopause Society and Women's Health Concern recommendations on hormone replacement therapy. Menopause Int. 2013;19:59–68.

    Pitkin J. Should HRT be duration limited? Menopause Int. 2013;19:167–74.
24. Brinton RD, Proffitt P, Tran J, et al. Equilin, a principal component of the estrogen replacement therapy Premarin, increases the

growth of cortical neurons via an NMDA receptor-dependent mechanism. Exp Neurol. 1997;147:211–20.

25. Bhavnani BR, Strickler RC. Menopausal hormone therapy. J Obstet Gynaecol Can. 2005;27:137–62.

26. Mehta et al., Risks, benefits, and treatment modalities.

27. Cappelleti M, Walen K. Increasing women's sexual desire: The comparative effectiveness of estrogens and androgens. Hormonal Behavior. 2016;78:178–93.

28. Parish SJ, Simon JA, Davis SR, et al. International Society for the Study of Women's Sexual Health Clinical Practice Guideline for the use of systemic testosterone for hypoactive sexual desire disorder in women. J Sexual Med. 2021;18:849–67.

29. Jayasena CN, Alkaabi FM, Liebers CS, et al. A systematic review of randomized controlled trials investigating the efficacy and safety of testosterone therapy for female sexual dysfunction in postmenopausal women. Clin Endocrinol. 2019;90:391–414.

30. Kaaks R, Berrino F, Key T, et al. Serum sex steroids in premenopausal women and breast cancer risk within the European prospective investigation into cancer and nutrition (EPIC). J Natl Cancer Inst. 2005;97:755–65.

Berrino F, Pasanisi P, Bellati C, et al. Serum testosterone levels and breast cancer recurrence. Int J Cancer. 2004;113:499–502.

31. Gera R, Tayeh S, Chihad He-H, et al. Does transdermal testosterone increase the risk of developing breast cancer? A systematic review. Anticancer Res. 2018;38:6615–20.

Glaser RL, York AE, Dimitrakakis C. Incidence of invasive breast cancer in women treated with testosterone implants: A prospective 10-year cohort study. BMC Cancer. 2019;19:1271.

32. Pickering G. Physician and scientist. BMJ. 1964,2:1615–19.

33. Blakemore C, Cooper GF. Development of the brain depends on the visual environment. Nature. 1970;228:477–78.

Index

INDEX

Hadler, Nortin M., 165
Halsted, William, 51
Hartz, Arthur, 139
*Harvard Medical School Health
    Letter,* 60
Healy, Bernadine, 6, 254
Healy, David, 139
Heart and Oestrogen/Progestin
    Replacement Study
    (HERS), 142
heart attacks, 132, 140; effects of
    statins, 145; mortality rate,
    147; nonfatal and fatal, 145;
    symptoms, 132–33
Hellman, Sam, 99
herbal supplements, 40–41
Hershman, Dawn, 100
Hill, Austin Bradford, 90,
    139–40, 195; causal
    relationship between agent
    and disease, 83–85; link
    between cigarette smoking
    and lung cancer, 85–86; link
    between oestrogen and breast
    cancer, 86–89
hip fractures, 152–54, 158, 161,
    167; benefit of oestrogen,
    158–59; bisphosphonates
    and, 166; calcium
    supplements for reducing,
    157; caused by osteoporosis,

152, 166; consequences, 155;
    drugs for, 167–68; effects of,
    153; impaired functioning
    and well-being from, 155;
    risk of death, 153–55
hippocampus, 184–85, 188
Hodis, Howard, 148
Holmberg, Lars, 119
Holtorf, Kent, 42
Hoover, Robert, 94
hormone replacement therapy
    (HRT), 4–5, 8–10, 30,
    48–49, 101–2, 105, 171, 192,
    215, 229–34, 255–57;
    advocacy, 24; alleviation of
    symptoms of depression, 33;
    association between breast
    cancer and, 57–61, 253;
    benefits, 6, 32, 129–30,
    149–50, 216, 234, 254;
    cardiovascular risk, 142;
    cognitive decline and, 91;
    cognitive functions and,
    179–81; deaths from breast
    cancer, 63–64; difference
    between antidepressants and,
    33–34; health-related
    quality of life, effect on, 14;
    menopausal symptoms,
    benefits on, 35–37; Million
    Women Study, 70–79;

osteoporosis and fractures, effect on, 158–59, 162–63; pilot study, 108–16; risk of dementia for women, 179, 181–82; risks of, 14–15, 73, 129–30, 245–46; risks *vs* benefits, 36; side effects and potential risks, 38; study of breast cancer survivors, 124–25; WHI's report, 61–70, 117

Hortobagyi, Gabriel N., 88

Hospital Adjustment Scale, 189

hot flushes, 28, 32; nonhormonal therapies for, 41

Huggins, Charles, 102

Hunter, David J., 221

Hupka, Barbara, 107

I

illusory correlations, 81–82

international menopause and women's health organizations, 242–43

Ioannidis, John, 237

Isoflavone Clover Extract Study, 40

J

James, Henry, 94

Jolie, Angelina, 135

Jordan, V. Craig, 88–89

Journal of Clinical Endocrinology and Metabolism, 38

Journal of the American Medical Association (JAMA): on HRT, 108–9, 239; on idalopirdine, 199; on statins, 146; on WHI study, 7–8, 65–67, 139

Journal of the North American Menopause Society, 225

K

Kahneman, Daniel, 236

Kantor, Herman, 189

Katz, Mitchell H., 146

Kennedy, Pagan, 174

Klingberg, Torkel, 202

Koch, Robert, 79; postulates, 79–82

Kolata, Gina, 27

Krumholz, Harlan, 147

L

Lancet, 60, 76, 91

Langer, Robert, 64, 166–67

Latina women, perimenopause symptoms, 29

lecanemab (Leqembi), 200

Legato, Marianne, 133; *The Female Heart,* 133

Lená, Sarah, 116

New York Times, 7, 24, 27, 48, 70, 158, 174, 221, 224
night sweats, 18, 30, 32, 35, 47, 101, 246
Niro, Robert De, 135
Nixon, Cynthia, 134
nonvertebral fractures, 163
North American Menopause Society, 7, 35–36, 43, 48, 241, 243
North American Menopause Society (NAMS), 243
Northrup, Dr. Christiane, 17
Notaro, Tig, 134
Nunn, Thomas William, 56
Nurses' Health Study, 77, 87, 137, 140, 142, 219

O
observational studies, 122, 149, 193, 238; on breast-conserving surgery, 52; on effects of HRT on breast cancer survivors, 116; nonrandomized, 139; randomized controlled trials compared to, 137–39; on risk of dementia, 208
obstructive coronary artery disease, 133

O'Donnell, Rosie, 135
oestrogen: benefits for brain, 186–89, 206–9; in birth control pills, 217; blood vessels, effect on, 142–43; brain's neuroplasticity and, 183; breast cancer and, 52–53, 55–61, 78, 86–89, 114–15, 128; cognitive functions and, 179, 185, 189–91, 207; deficiency symptoms, 25; dementia and, 207, 209; endogenous, 136; heart health and, 136–37, 149; level in women after menopause, 183; platelet clumping, 143; plus progesterone, benefits, 56–57; during pregnancy, 53–55, 103; prevention of osteoporosis, 156, 158–59; product warning, 14; risk of hip fractures, 159–60, 167; risk of stroke, 192–96; therapy, 4; vaginal, 225–26; WHI warning on preparations of, 117
O'Meara, Ellen, 116, 126
omega 3s, 40
oncology, 97
oral contraceptives, 217–24

osteoid, 155

osteomalacia, 156

osteopenia, 158, 164–65;
 diagnosis, 164

osteoporosis, 151–52, 156, 158,
 160–61, 170; calcium and
 vitamins, role of, 156–57;
 development, 152; preventive
 treatment of, 165–66; sign
 of advanced, 153; in
 women, 152

Our Bodies, Ourselves, 23

ovarian cancer, 58

ovarian cancers, 219–20

ovarian failure, 27

P

Palshof, Torben, 103

Parker-Pope, Tara, 63; *The
 Hormone Decision,* 21

Partridge, Ann, 54

Patinkin, Mandy, 135

Patnaik, Jennifer, 135

Pearson, Cynthia, 24, 26

perimenopause, 13, 19

Peters, George, 115

Peto, Richard, 61

Petretta, Mario, 145–46

PET scans of brain, 187

Phillips, Stuart, 190

Pickering, Sir George White, 251

Pignone, Michael, 145

Pike, Malcolm, 229

Poggio, Francesca, 127

Postmenopausal Oestrogen/
 Progestin Interventions trial
 (PEPI), 137

postmenopausal osteoporosis,
 156–57

postmenopausal women, 39;
 BRCA1 and BRCA2
 mutations, 58; cognitive
 ability, 176, 206, 208;
 effect of exercise, 162–63,
 170–71; oestrogen and
 progesterone therapy, 104;
 oestrogen-deficiency
 symptoms, 25; hip fractures
 in, 154; hormone
 replacement therapy, 6, 32,
 66, 93; hormone replacement
 therapy benefits, 112, 122,
 137, 150, 159, 171, 178;
 incidence of heart attacks
 and cardiac deaths, 140–41;
 MPA treatment, 213;
 osteoporosis in, 156, 167–69;
 osteoporotic fractures in,
 158; risk of breast cancer, 59,
 104, 107; risk of stroke, 193;
 romosozumab therapy, 169

Pott, Percivall, 83

Powell, Colin, 135

prefrontal cortex, 184

About the Authors

Avrum Bluming received his MD from the Columbia College of Physicians and Surgeons. He spent four years as a senior investigator for the National Cancer Institute and for two of those years was director of the Lymphoma Treatment Center in Kampala, Uganda. He organized the first study of lumpectomy for the treatment of breast cancer in Southern California in 1978, and for more than two decades he has been studying the benefits and risks of hormone replacement therapy administered to women with a history of breast cancer. Dr. Bluming has served as a clinical professor of medicine at USC and has been an invited speaker at the Royal College of Physicians in London and the Pasteur Institute in Paris. He was elected to mastership in the American College of Physicians, an honor accorded to only five hundred of the over one hundred thousand board-certified internists in this country.

Carol Tavris received her PhD in social psychology from the University of Michigan. Her books include *Mistakes Were Made (but Not by Me)*, with Elliot Aronson; *Anger: The Misunderstood Emotion;* and *The Mismeasure of Woman.* She has written articles, op-eds, and book reviews on topics in psychological science for a wide array of publications—including the *Los Angeles Times,* the *New York Times Book Review,* the *Wall Street Journal,* and the *Times Literary Supplement*—and a column for *Skeptic* magazine. She is a fellow of the Association for Psychological Science and has received numerous awards for her efforts to promote gender equality, science, and skepticism.